FAMILY
SECRETS
THE BEST OF THE DELTA

Lee Academy
Clarksdale, Mississippi

Lee Academy is a college preparatory school which provides an educational environment of excellence with high academic and behavioral standards. The school nurtures the growth of the individual student with regard to specific needs and abilities in an atmosphere of warmth and care. A further purpose is to develop strong character in each student by teaching principles of self-discipline, respect for authority, patriotism, a love of learning, and a reverence for God.

Additional copies of Family Secrets may be obtained by using the order form at the back of the book or writing:

Family Secrets
Lee Academy
415 Lee Drive
Clarksdale, Mississippi   38614

Please enclose your return address with a check payable to Family Secrets in the amount of $14.95 plus $2.50 postage and handling. Mississippi residents add $1.05 sales tax per book.

First Edition, First Printing, 6,000 copies, October 1990
Second Printing, 5,000 copies, January 1993

Copyright 1990
Lee Academy
Clarksdale, Mississippi

Library of Congress Card Catalog 90-060225
ISBN 0-9626151 - 0 - 2

Printed in the USA by
WIMMER BROTHERS
A Wimmer Company
Memphis • Dallas

CONTENTS

COMMITTEE

Chairman	Emily Cooper
Design	Meg Agostinelli Margie Cooper
Recipes	Roselyn Dulaney
Typing	Peggy Beckham Betty Lynn Hunt
Marketing	Sue Bell Jennie Neblett
Business	Linda Dulaney

PHOTOGRAPHY

The Lee Academy Cookbook Committee is grateful to Chuck Lamb for the donation of his time and talent.

Chuck Lamb, Owner of Lamb's Photography, Clarksdale, Mississippi, has achieved a high level of photographic excellence as evidenced not only by the numerous awards and prestigious degrees he has earned, but also by the demand of his services by regional, state and local professional photographic associations.

He studied photography extensively during undergraduate years and has continued his studies ever since. After establishing his own studio in 1982, he has been continually recognized for his highly interpretive style of photography. He has earned the Mississippi and National Certified Photographers Degree, the Mississippi Service Degree and the Mississippi Photographer of the Year Award.

We want to sincerely thank all those who contributed their time and talent to this cookbook. Without them it would not have been possible.

Abraham, William	Flowers, Graydon	Luster, Fisher
Agostinelli, Thomas	Flowers, Mr. and Mrs. Graydon	Maclin, Patsy
Allen, Mary Wilsford	Flowers, Mr. and Mrs. Harry	Marley, Gayla
Allen, Rita	Flowers, Scott	Marley, Minette
Antici, Beverly	Fong, Cindy	Mc Cullough, Ms. Jenny
Bailey, Jason	Foster, Carla	Mc Dowell, Mrs. Margurite
Balducci, Jill	Foster, Lesley	Mc Murchy, Caroline
Boyd, Mrs. Hazel	Foster, Mrs. Frank	Mc Murchy, Mrs. Betty
Bradham, Jo Ann	Foster, Shelley	Meredith, Pam
Bramlett, Mrs. Medora	Fowler, Kathy	Merkel, Charles
Bratschi, Janet	Frazer, Penny	Middleton, Clint
Britt, Mr. and Mrs. Freddie	Fyfe, Brian	Mitchell, Pam
Burkes, Ms. Mildred	Gamble, Wanda	Monty, Mrs. Charles Sr.
Butler, Allison	Garrison, Rod	Murphey, Sylvia
Campbell, Elizabeth	Gates, Lynn	Murray, Brian
Carlson, Chrissy	Glidewell, Allison	Neblett, Mr. and Mrs. Rives
Chamoun, Ms. Vivian	Goss, Mary Virginia	Olson, Nancy
Chow, Alice	Grant, Beverly	Parolli, Jason
Chow, Sally	Grant, Mr. and Mrs. Gerry	Parsons, Carlisle
Cohen, Stuart	Graves, Barbara	Phillips, Kristen
Connell, Mr. and Mrs. Ed	Graves, Matt	Poole, Mary
Connell, Ted	Harden,, William	Poole, Meredith
Cooper, Jean	Hatchett, Meg	Redner, Michelle
Cooper, John	Hirsberg, Jodi	Seymore, Manda
Cooper, Mr. and Mrs. Tom	Hite, Lynn	Sigmon, Mr. and Mrs. Marvin
Craig, Chism	Houston, Brian	Sims, Mr. and Mrs. Tommy
Crook, Tripp	Houston, Susan	Smith, Art
Davis, Amie	Hussey, Anne	Stringer, Carolyn
Davis, Carolyn	Hussey, Annesley	Surholt, Mr. and Mrs. Fred
Dilworth, Mary	Hussey, Curry	Thompson, Mary
Donald, Sherry	Hussey, Edwin	Townsend, Judy
Duff, Jean	Jacob, Rachael	Tyner, Maggie
Dulaney, Mr. and Mrs. Edwin	Kittell, Mr. and Mrs. Dean	Tyner, Mimi
Dunn, Rachel	Kittle, Lynn	Webb, Carolyn
Eason, Sherry	Laney, Johnny	Websteer, Richard
Fiser, Mrs. Hal	Longino, Jane	Wilson, Georgia
Flowers, Amelia	Longino, Johnny	Wilson, Jim
Flowers, Charles	Longino, Mrs. John T.	Wise, John
Flowers, Gay	Longino, Reed	Youngblood, Mrs. Regina

HEALTH SECRETS

When our Mississippi Delta families get together, feasting is an age-old tradition. From Thanksgiving dinner once a year to Sunday lunch at Grandmother's once a week, food is a part of the pleasure of such occasions. As much as we enjoy them, many of these cherished recipes have traditionally been high in fat and salt. However, we can not ignore the advice of a growing number of health experts that a diet high in fat and sodium can contribute to disease conditions, particularly cancer and heart disease. So, is it necessary to give these foods up altogether to eat a healthy diet? Hardly! The following are some tips that can be applied to your general cooking that will help you have a lower-fat, lower - sodium lifestyle. Also, throughout the entire book we have added recipe adaptations.

• Eat a variety of foods everyday. That is, two servings (3 ounces) of meat or fish, two glasses of low fat dairy products, four servings of fruits and vegetables and four grain foods.

• Choose lean cuts of meat and poultry. Trim outside fat; remove skin before cooking.

• Tenderize lean cuts by marinating, cubing, or mechanically tenderizing.

• Eat smaller servings of higher-fat meats, desserts and appetizers.

• Rely on herbs and spices for seasoning rather than salt, butter, margarine, heavy sauces or gravies.

• Use lower-fat substitutes for traditional high-fat items. Example: Substitute plain low-fat yogurt for sour cream or use a mix of low-fat cottage and light cream cheese - based spreads or dips.

• Reduce by one half the amount of fat called for in a recipe. The microwave is a great help in streaming without fat.

• Decrease the amount of high-fat meats and cheeses by half and increase the amount of starch or vegetable to give the same volume.

• Always skim the excess fat from broths and stews. Do this by chilling the broth or soup; the fat will rise to the top.

• Festive foods aren't the only aspect of entertaining. Focus on the decor, the music, and most of all, the people.

Emily M. Cooper, R.D., L.D.

FOREWORD

The Lee Academy Cookbook Collection is a unique treasure. When asked to write the foreward, I gave warning that had they scoured the countryside, they could not have chosen one with fewer culinary skills. My only claim to fame is a Hot Hershey Sandwich—only because no one in these parts had ever heard of it.

Some twenty-eight years ago we moved to Mississippi and were amazed to discover that Clarksdale women were great cooks. I was somehow of the opinion that Southern ladies needed a road map to find their way to the kitchen where the family cook presided. I soon learned that they not only could cook—many were in the gourmet class, as you will discover when you try some of the great recipes in this book.

In addition to the traditional Southern cooking Clarksdale is blessed with many ethnic groups who grace this book with an abundance of exciting recipes.

Wyatt Cooper, in his delightful book, *Families* wrote—"They say the family is finished, but I don't believe it!" He cherished the memory of early family reunions and the exchange of favorite recipes, just as Clarksdalians remember their families and their heritage, including the sharing of skills from Grandmother's kitchen. Bon Appetite!

Mary Jo McIntosh

Christmas Cookies

Can't you just smell the cinnamon
and nutmeg? What a happy way for
families to share in the preparation
of holiday foods. That is what family
traditions are all about - passing
down from generation to generation, not only the secret recipes, but
the love!

*Fix some Christmas treats for your spe-
cial family. Try Chocolate Star Peanut
Butter Cookies (Page 222) with Icing
(Page 205) and Buttermilk Pralines
(Page 242).*

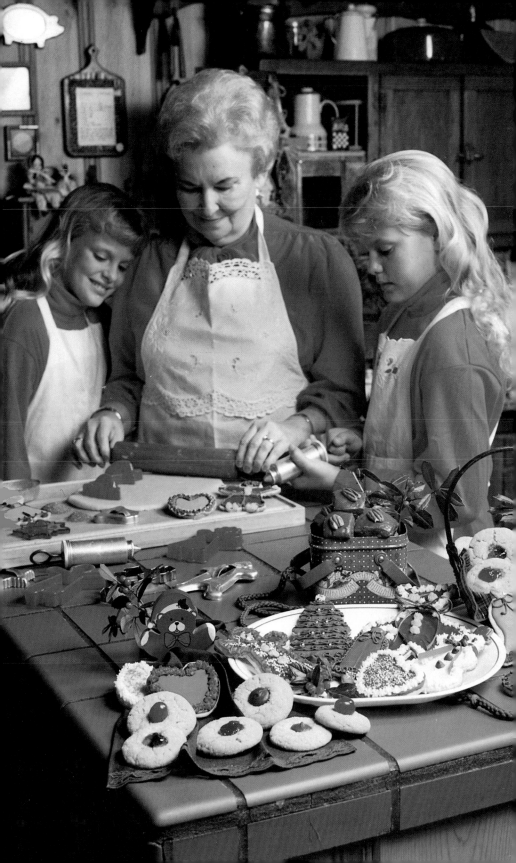

Play Lady Party

One of the oldest and most precious traditions in a little girl's life is her "Play Lady Party". The fun of rummaging through Grandmama's high heeled shoes, hats and gloves is truly an exciting time. A "Play Lady Party" is a very special occasion, and more important, it is an on-going example that the art of being a good hostess can never start too soon.

No Banana Split is complete without Jane's Hot Fudge Sauce (Page 248).

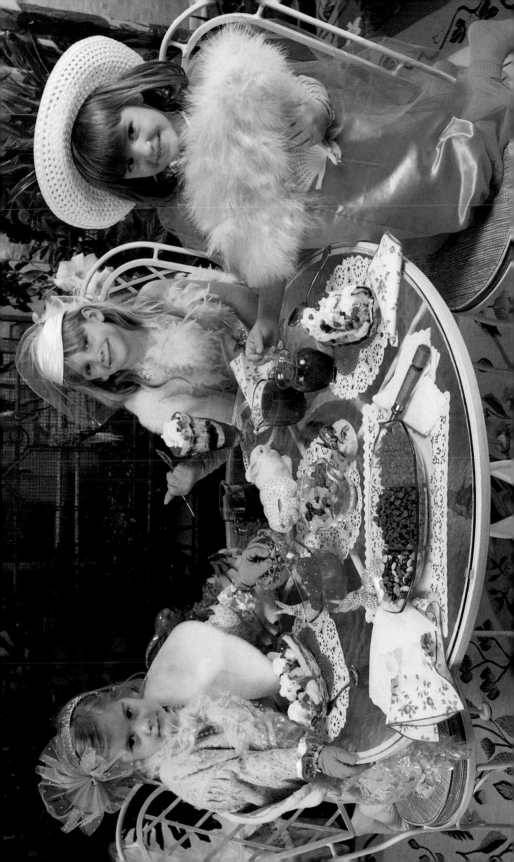

Tennis

What a fun way to spend an afternoon! Good friends, a close tennis match, and an array of appetizing dips and spreads. Nothing hits the spot better than a tall glass of iced tea and a tasty "Pick up" food. Surprise your guests with the results of your favorite recipes, and they will always come back for more.

It's time to take a break and enjoy Shrimp Bites In Puff Pastry (Page 44), Charles Cheese Spread (Page 33) with fresh vegetables, Citrus Tea (Page 50) and Pineapple Dip With Fruit (Page 37).

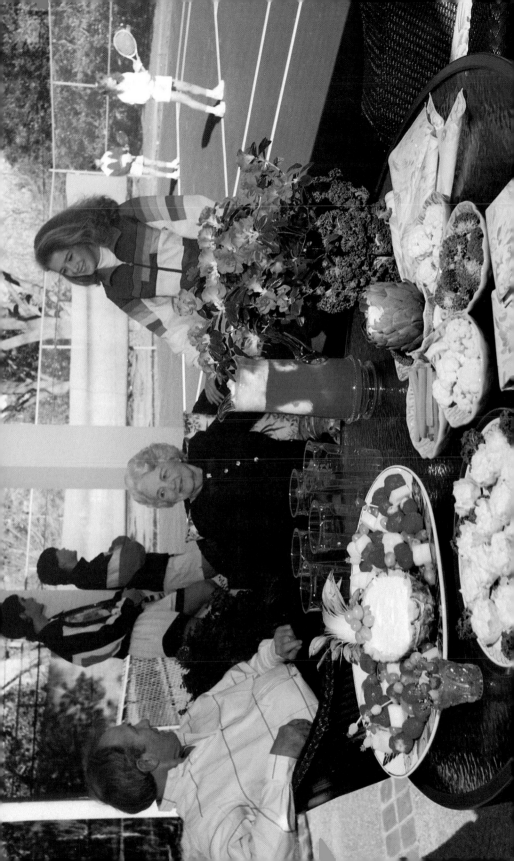

Pasta

We all know that the best thing that ever happened to America was Columbus. But the next best thing was Italian pasta! On a cold winter night nothing tastes better than a plate of spaghetti swimming in tomato-meat sauce and covered with freshly grated Parmesan cheese. Or what about a dish of little pillows of meat? Not the frozen-food kind, but ravioli that has been made from scratch in someone's kitchen. The dish selections are endless. Fettucini, Cappelletti, and Lasagna! All are hearty and zesty, and they all are made from closely guarded family secrets.

Ravioli (Page 114) and Spaghetti With Meat Sauce (Page 111) are favorite pasta dishes.

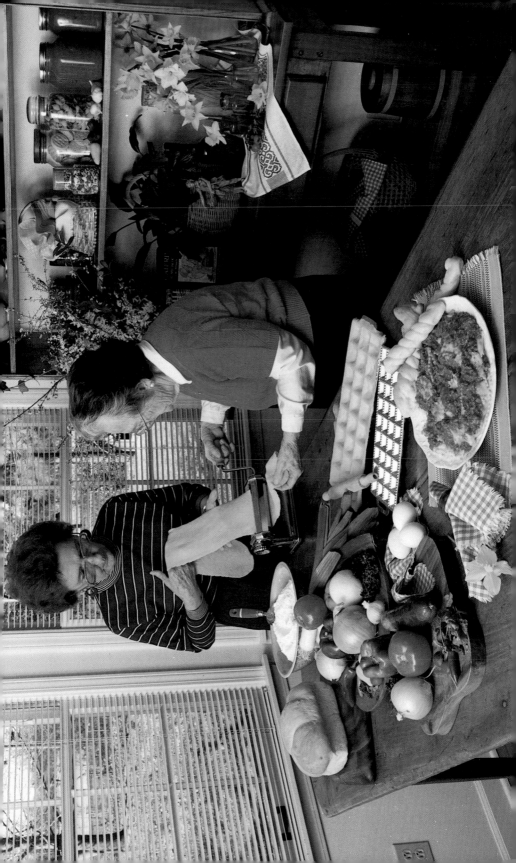

Levee

The levee has always played an important part in the lives of all the people in our area. This man-made dike not only holds back the Mighty Mississippi, it also affords a perfect place for an outing on a crisp autumn afternoon. The levee is an ideal setting for the bountiful spread of a typical Delta "Everybody Bring Something" picnic.

Our Levee Picnic is overflowing with goodies - Jack-O-Lantern Pumpkin Bread (Page 96), Oven Fried Sesame Chicken (Page 136), Mint Tea (Page 50), Baked Bean Medley (Page 180) and sour dough bread along with buckets full of fall fruit.

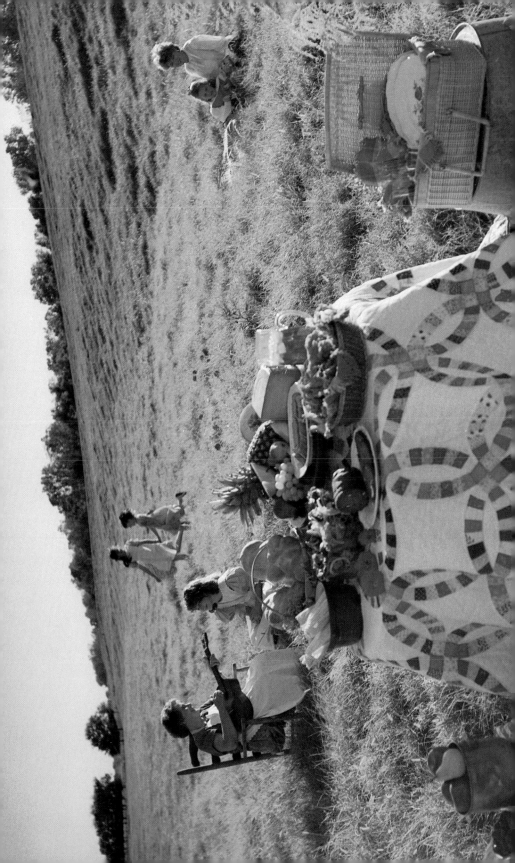

Chow

What would a Delta wedding be without a bride's cake made by Sally and Alice Chow? Their finished products are truly works of art for the eyes and delights to the palates of all who appreciate perfection. They have started their own tradition, one to be added to the many other customs of their heritage. Food has always played an important role in all Chinese celebrations, and now the Chow cakes will take their place among these time-honored rituals.

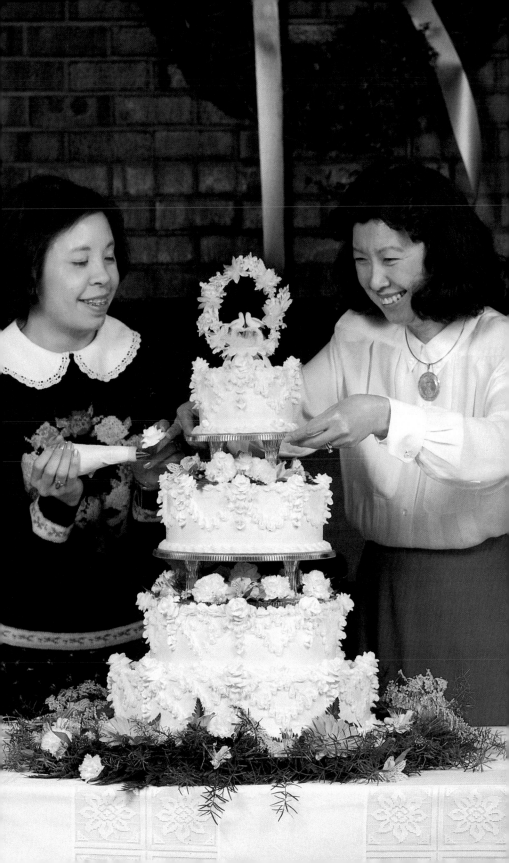

Thanksgiving

Is there anything more wonderful than watching Grandaddy carve the Thanksgiving turkey? The harvest table is groaning under the weight of dishes of dressing, vegetables, and fruits. The platters of hot, homemade rolls are dripping with butter. The sideboard is laden with desserts of every description - and once again, a family can come together to give thanks for all its blessings.

A Thanksgiving feast wouldn't be complete without Woody's Rolls (Page 100), Grandmother Freeman's Sweet Potato Casserole (Page 183) and Ma Brewer's Cuban Flan (Page 239).

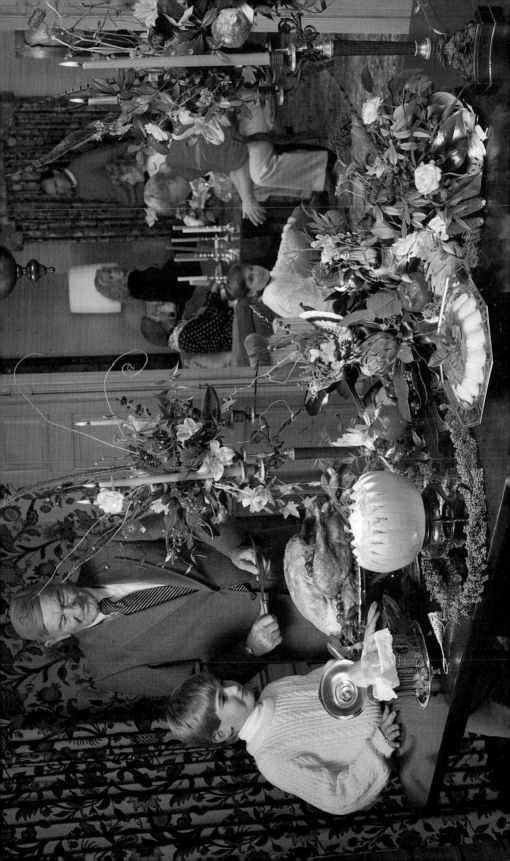

Chamoun's Grocery

In every town there will always be one favorite eating place where friends meet comfortably to have lunch and talk over the crops, the children and world affairs. Chamoun's Grocery is such a place! When celebrities or foreign trade boards come for a visit, the first meal they usually have is at this small store. Although many good foods are offered on the menu, most guests choose the Lebanese kibbie, cabbage rolls and salad. All of these dishes are made from authentic Lebanese recipes that are and have been the Chamouns' family secrets.

Lunch today is Kibbie (Page 107) and French Fries.

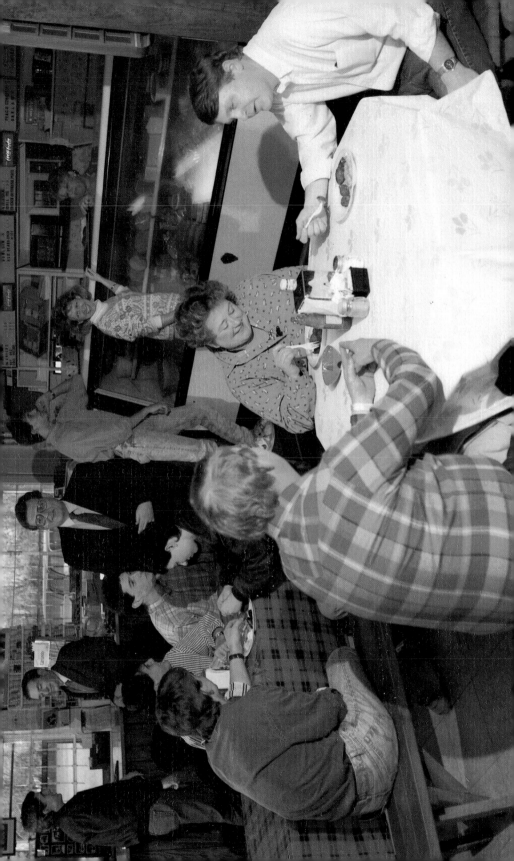

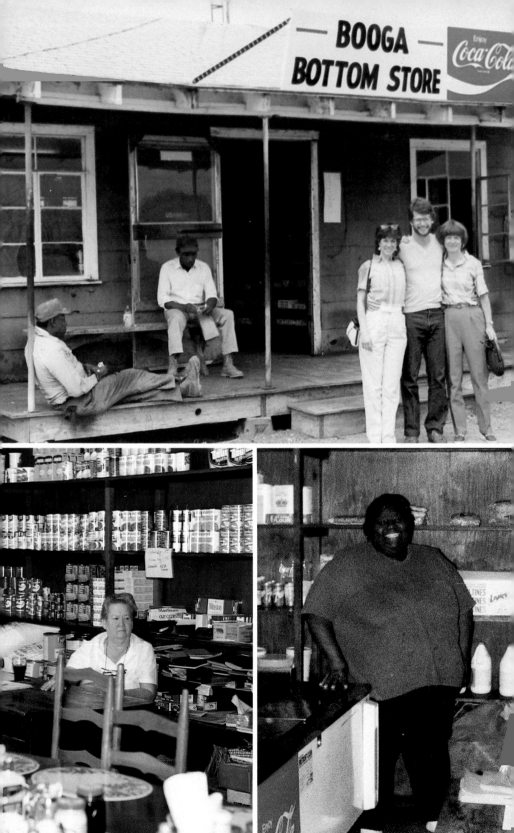

Booga Bottom

Set out to find the pot of gold at the end of the rainbow, and if you are lucky, you will find Booga Bottom Store. This priceless jewel is set in the middle of rice and soybean fields — not easy to find, but well worth the effort. Inside are one large and two small tables covered with oilcloth. Then you see Margarite McDowell who has run this amazing cafe since 1969, and Mildred Burks (fondly known as "Teddy Bear") who has been the cook all these years. There are no menus; soul food is served up in the manner of plantation plate lunches. Entrées can range from meatloaf to chicken and dumplings, and the fresh vegetables are unlimited. Delicious cornbread, biscuits, or rolls accompany the meal. When you think you can't eat another bite, out come homemade pies, piping hot from the oven. This is really living — Southern style!

CHINESE GUEST MENU

Red is a traditional Chinese color and should be used frequently at the table in the china and linens.

Egg Drop Soup (Page 66)

Egg Rolls (Page 120)

Sweet and Sour Chicken Wings (Page 133)

Broccoli with Beef (Page 117)

Shrimp Cantonese (Page 161)

Steamed Rice

Fortune Cookies

Hot Tea

ITALIAN SUPPER

Antipasto: Salami and Proscuitto

Black Olives and Marinated Artichoke Hearts

Bread Sticks

Duck Stufato on Gnocchi (Page 151)

Green Salad with Italian Dressing (Page 90)

Italian Dressing Bread (Page 93)

Ma Brewer's Cuban Flan (Page 239)

MAD HATTER'S TEA PARTY

Schedule this little girls birthday party or ladies tea for the month of April. Decorate the table with festive hats and flowers in the center. The invitation should encourage the wearing of a spring hat. Little girls should dress as characters from *Alice in Wonderland*.

Tea Cakes (Page 229)

Jam Cookies (Page 223)

Chess Squares (Page 224)

Peanut Butter Balls (Page 244)

Cathy's Famous Christmas Fudge (Page 242)

Sara Jane's Toffee (Page 243)

Individual Cheese Cakes (Page 201)

Orange Sunshine (Page 51)

EASTER FAMILY BRUNCH

NOON

Have an Easter egg hunt before the meal for the children. Decorate the table with Easter bunnies of all kinds and shapes. Intersperse white Dogwood branches throughout. The centerpiece is a large Easter egg tree with each child's name on an ornament.

Turkey Hash in Pastry Shells (Page 147)

Butter Coffee Cakes (Page 95)

Soufflé of Grits (Page 55)

Frittata (Italian Spinach and Eggs) (Page 187)

Applesauce Salad (Page 87)

Crème Brulée (Page 234)

FORMAL DINNER PARTY

A BIRTHDAY CELEBRATION

Have gold balloons tied to the guest of honor's chair. One big helium balloon is at his plate with champagne and a gag gift inside. Flowers are pale peach amaryllis. Mirror tiles with votive candles placed in the center are interspersed along the entire table. To begin the meal, guests gather around the table and the honoree is given a large hat pin. When he pops the balloon present, the first course is brought — a very effective way to start dinner with a "Bang"!

Soup   Cheesy Broccoli Bisque (Page 60)

Fish   Catfish in Shells (Page 156)

Salad   Spinach Salad with Dressing (Page 82)

Sorbet   Three Fruit Sherbet (Page 245)

Entreé   Butterflied Leg of Lamb (Page 130)

Rice Supreme (Page 171)

Fresh Asparagus Bundles Tied with Lemon Rind

Jenny's Herb Rolls (Page 102)

Dessert Scrumptious Apricot Soufflé (Page 230)

FAMILY CHRISTMAS DINNER

Have the dining table set with personalized Christmas ornaments at each place. Children under seven usually enjoy sitting at a little table to the side. Everyone loves finding a small Christmas gift on each plate. Have festive holiday music playing and enjoy the warmth and good food. After dinner everyone gathers around the tree to open more gifts and sing. Read the Biblical Christmas Story and *The Night Before Christmas*.

Baked Dove Breasts on Toast Points (Page 150)

Easy Hot Fruit (Page 176)

Evelyn's Cornbread Dressing (Page 172)

Asparagus Casserole (Page 177)

Hot Rolls (Page 93)

Puffed Pastry Filled with Green Boiled Custard (Page 235)

You can buy the pastry from the freezer section at the grocery. Cut it with Christmas tree cookie cutter. Pull out the center but leave bottom. Bake.

VALENTINE DINNER FOR TWO

Set the table with a red table cloth and white napkins. Put a gift on the table for your sweetheart and Valentines cards on each plate. Use champagne glasses with decorative, glitter fun-sticks from the florist coming out on the top. Have the wine cooler with Champagne iced nearby.

Broccoli Soup (Page 61)

Stuffed Chicken Breasts Savannah (Page 142)

Eggplant Casserole (Page 183)

Scalloped Potatoes (Page 186)

Vanilla Ice Cream with Raspberry Sauce (Page 236)

Robert E. Lee Cookies (Page 229)

DELTA BLUES PARTY

Set up the yard like a festival with colorful booths. The booths are several individual tables covered with bright oilcloth under large signs advertising "Shrimp", "Crawfish" and "Oysters". Have seafood iced in large serving bowls accompanied by sauces on each table. Have a longer buffet table for the remaining food nearby covered in colorful burlap. The centerpiece is cotton bolls, milo, alfalfa, wheat and other fall foilage. Have a Blues Combo. Attire for the event is casual. Enclose a bandana in the invitation and tell each guest to wear it to the party.

Pork Tenderloin with Barbeque Sauce (Page 124)

Remoulade Sauce (Page 193)

Booga Bottom Turnips (Page 189)

Sweet Potato Casserole (Page 183)

Grandmother's Cornbread (Page 97)

Stewed Tomatoes and Okra

New Years Blackeyed Peas (Page 181)

Easy Fresh Peach Cobbler (Page 213)

Mom's Pound Cake (Page 208)

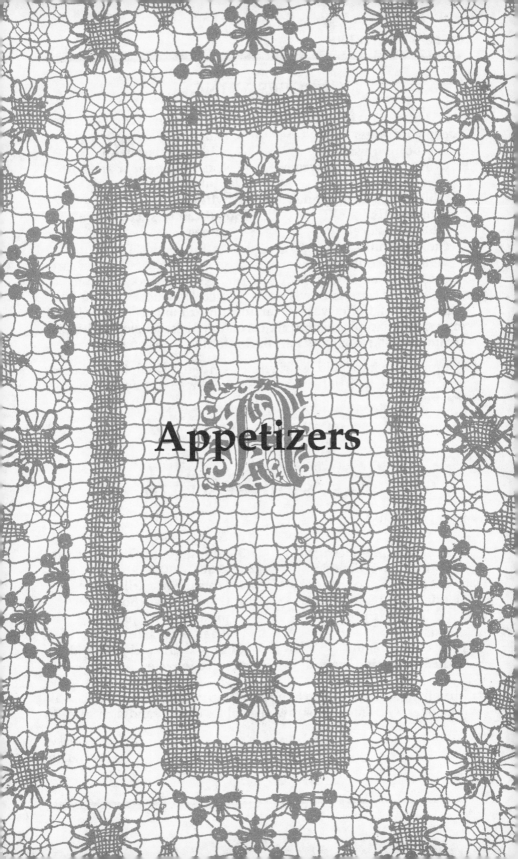

Appetizers

CHEESE RING

1½ packages plain gelatin
¼ cup cold water
¼ cup boiling water
6 (3 ounce) packages cream
  cheese
3 tablespoons bell pepper,
  chopped fine
3 tablespoons celery,
  chopped fine
3 tablespoons onion,
  chopped fine

2 tablespoons Worcestershire
  sauce
2 tablespoons catsup
  Dash red pepper and salt
½ pint whipping cream,
  whipped
Small can of sliced green
  olives

Soak gelatin in cold water 5 minutes. Add boiling water. Mix all ingredients except whipped cream in order listed. Fold in whipped cream. Oil ring mold and garnish bottom with sliced green olives.

Pour mixture into mold. Refrigerate overnight. Unmold just before serving. Serve with butter crackers. Great for a reception or tea. Can not freeze.

Verne Kittell
Clarksdale

CARY'S CHEESE SPREAD

YIELD: 6 CUPS

4 (8 ounce) pre-packaged
  grated sharp Cheddar
  cheese
16 ounces mayonnaise
3 tablespoons prepared
  mustard
Juice of one lemon
¼ medium onion, grated

3 tablespoons Worcestershire
  sauce
1 tablespoon garlic salt
1 (2 ounce) jar chopped
  pimento with juice
Hot sauce to taste
Chopped green chilies and
  juice to taste

Mix all ingredients well in large bowl with mixer or by hand. Use as appetizer with crackers or raw vegetables or as a sandwich spread.

Cary Cocke
Clarksdale

CHARLES CHEESE BALL

SERVES: A BUNCH

2 (8 ounce packages) cream cheese
1 bunch green onions, chopped fine
½ teaspoon monosodium glutamate

1 jar dried beef, chopped fine
1 teaspoon salt - optional
1 cup chopped black olives
Chopped pecans

Soften cream cheese. Mix all ingredients and roll in chopped pecans.

Alice Lee Hayes
Clarksdale

PINEAPPLE CHEESE BALLS

YIELD: 3 MEDIUM SIZE BALLS

2 (8 ounce) packages cream cheese, softened
1 (8½ ounce) cans crushed pineapple, drained
¼ cup chopped bell pepper

2 tablespoons minced onion
1 tablespoon seasoned salt
Few drops red hot sauce
2 cups chopped pecans

Combine all ingredients, except 1 cup of chopped pecans. Roll in balls, chill, then roll in remaining cup of pecans.

Margaret Keeler
Clarksdale

CHEESE STRAWS

YIELD: 4 DOZEN   OVEN: 425

1 pound extra sharp Cheddar cheese
½ pound butter, softened

3 cups plain flour
1 teaspoon salt
½ teaspoon red pepper

Grate cheese. Let cheese get very soft. Mix with butter. Gradually add flour mixed with salt and pepper. Mix well. Put through cookie press using "star" point. Bake on cookie sheet (sprayed lightly with cooking spray) for 6 to 8 minutes or until lightly brown.

Verne Kittell
Clarksdale

HERBED CHEESE DOLLARS

YIELD: 6 DOZEN   OVEN: 400°

¼ cup margarine, softened
½ pound sharp Cheddar
  cheese, grated
1¼ cups all-purpose flour
  (measured before sifting)
¼ teaspoon dried basil

¼ teaspoon ground sage
¼ teaspoon powered thyme
3 shakes cayenne pepper
2 tablespoons dry white
  wine

Combine margarine and cheese; beat until thoroughly blended. Add other ingredients and form into a long roll about the size of a silver dollar. Wrap in waxed paper and chill until firm. To bake, slice ⅛ inch thick and place on lightly greased baking sheet and bake 10 minutes. Store in airtight container. Freezes beautifully.

Peggy Beckham
Clarksdale

CHUTNEY CHEESE PATÉ

SERVES: 20 TO 25

MOLD:
1 (8 ounce) package cream
  cheese, softened
1 cup grated sharp Cheddar
  cheese

4 tablespoons sherry
1 teaspoon curry powder
¼ teaspoon salt

Combine cheeses, sherry, curry powder, and salt. Mix well in food processor until creamy and smooth. Pour into spring form pan and press to a smooth mold, about ½ inch thick. Chill. (Best if made a day before)

TOPPING:
1 cup chutney
½ cup shredded coconut

½ cup green onions, chopped
½ cup chopped peanuts

Before serving, spoon chutney on top. Add a layer of chopped green onions, a layer of chopped peanuts and a layer of coconut. If you prefer, you can garnish in rings of onions, peanuts and coconut rather than layers. Remove the sides of the spring pan and place the cheese mold on a serving tray. Circle with crackers.

Mrs. Clifford Davis
Clarksdale

CHILI MACHO

From the Rio de Balanos to bayous of eastern Arkansas and now to the Yazoo Delta comes this salsa which has left a hot trail enroute.

SERVES: 6

1 clove of garlic, minced
1 medium purple onion, chopped
1 (16 ounce) can tomatoes, chopped
3 fresh tomatoes, peeled and chopped
3 to 4 fresh jalepeño peppers, seeded and chopped, or 2 cans of jalepeños

1 teaspoon of salt
½ teaspoon cayenne
½ teaspoon of oregeno
1 teaspoon chili powder
½ teaspoon of cumin
½ teaspoon of cilantro

Combine all ingredients and refrigerate for 8 hours. Serve with tortilla chips.

The Phantom of the Delta - Lowell Taylor
Hughes, Arkansas

HUMAS DIP

SERVES: 10-12

2 (15 ounce) cans garbanzo beans, drained
Salt
1 cup tahini (sesame butter)
Juice of 6 fresh lemons or equivalent in substitute

2 peeled cloves garlic (if less garlic is desired, use 1 teaspoon chopped garlic or 2 teaspoons garlic powder)

Place all ingredients in a food processor and blend until mixture is a thick, smooth consistency. Add salt to taste and more lemon if desired. Place on platter and garnish with paprika and fresh mint or parsley. Chill before serving. Use as an appetizer spread on crackers, pita bread, or raw vegetables.

Family Secret: Sesame butter can usually be found in health food stores or in imported food sections of supermarkets. It is a common food in the Middle East and is used in much the way mayonnaise is used in America. This food is high in protein and an excellent dish for persons who are unable to tolerate dairy products.

Louise Chamoun
Clarksdale

EGGPLANT WITH SESAME OIL
(BABA GHANOUJ)

SERVES: 6

1 medium eggplant, dark-
   skinned (pierced with fork
   to let steam escape)
1 to 2 cloves garlic
Salt to taste
3 tablespoons sesame oil
Juice of 2 lemons

2 tablespoons water
2 tablespoons pine nuts
   (optional)
2 tablespoons pomegranate
   seeds (optional)
2 tablespoons chopped
   parsley

Broil eggplant, leaving skin on, on grill, turning frequently. Remove skin under cold water and mash eggplant. Pound garlic with salt; add sesame oil, lemon juice and water. Then mix with eggplant and salt. Spread on a platter and garnish with fresh parsley. Can also be garnished with pine nuts and pomegranate seeds.

Family Secret: Serve with crackers or use pita or pocket bread that has been cut in triangles then toasted slowly in low temperature oven. Best if served on a bland cracker. Sesame oil can be purchased in Clarksdale at Chamoun's Grocery and can be left in refrigerator indefinitely. It can also be purchased at Middle Eastern food stores, in Memphis at Barzizza Brothers or in Vicksburg at George M. Nassour.

Georgia Wilson
Clarksdale

CUCUMBER DIP

SERVES: 12

1 cup unpeeled, grated
   cucumber
2 (8 ounce) packages of
   cream cheese
1 tablespoon Worcestershire
   sauce

2 tablespoons grated onion
3 tablespoons mayonnaise
Dash of salt, pepper,
   monosodium glutamate
2 tablespoons lemon juice

Drain all the "water" from the cucumber making certain there is no moisture left in it. Mix all ingredients in blender and chill. Serve with corn chips.

Susan Connell
Clarksdale

PINEAPPLE DIP

SERVES: 2 CUPS

1 (8 ounce) package cream
   cheese, softened
½ (6 ounce) can frozen orange
   juice thawed

1 (8 ounce) can crushed
   pineapple, drained
1 (7 ounce) jar marshmallow
   creme

Mix cream cheese, pineapple, and marshmallow creme. Pour orange juice gradually into above mixture so that mixture will be thick enough to dip mixed fresh fruit. This dip is especially good with fresh strawberries.

Evelyn Harris
Lyon

CHICKEN LOG

SERVES: 12

2 (8 ounce) packages cream
   cheese, softened
1 tablespoon steak sauce
½ to 1 teaspoon curry powder
1½ cups minced chicken

⅓ cup minced celery
¼ cup chopped parsley
¼ cup chopped toasted
   almonds

Beat together first three ingredients. Blend in next 2 ingredients plus 2 tablespoons parsley. Shape mixture into log. Wrap in plastic wrap and chill 4 hours, or overnight. Toss together remaining parsley and almonds. Use to coat log. Serve with crackers.

Georgia Haaga
Clarksdale

SALMON SPREAD

SERVES:6

1 cup mayonnaise
1 dill pickle, chopped fine
Lemon juice

½ small onion, chopped fine
1 (15½ ounce) can salmon

Mix first four ingredients and let sit overnight in refrigerator. Spread 1 can salmon over a tray. Pour mixture over the salmon and serve with crackers.

Margaret Keeler
Clarksdale

SMOKED CATFISH MOUSSE

When our son Ross became a catfish farmer, I decided it was time to promote Mississippi catfish. For a Christmas party, I introduced this different way to use this delicious product which has become such a vital part of Mississippi.

SERVES: 20 TO 25

1 beef bouillon cube
1 cup boiling water
1 package gelatin
2 tablespoons cold water
2 tablespoons lemon juice
4 cups smoked catfish, minced (about 8 fillets)
4 tablespoons mayonnaise

1 (8 ounce package) cream cheese
Hot Sauce to taste (about ¼ teaspoon)
3 tablespoons grated onion
Salt to taste (about ½ teaspoon)

Dissolve bouillon in boiling water. Dissolve gelatin in cold water. Put gelatin mixture in bouillon and dissolve. Stir in lemon juice and fish. Add all other ingredients and beat with a wire whisk until smooth. Spray a 1½ to 2 - quart mold (preferably fish mold) with cooking spray. Add catfish mixture and refrigerate. When congealed, unmold. If you have used a fish mold, garnish with an olive slice for the eye and parsley around base, also paprika across back. Serve with your favorite crackers.

Family Secret: Smoke catfish on your water smoker. This takes about 1½ hours. This can be done at any time. Whenever you are smoking something else just put a few catfish fillets with it. Take off after 1½ hours. Crumble and freeze if you don't plan to make this right away.

Harvey Fiser
Clarksdale

SHRIMP BALL

1 (7½ ounce) can shrimp, drained and chopped
1 (8 ounce) package cream cheese, softened
2 tablespoons grated onion
3 teaspoons horseradish

2 teaspoons red hot sauce
1 teaspoon salt
1 tablespoon chopped green pepper
Chopped pecans

CONTINUED, SHRIMP BALL

Combine first seven ingredients, mixing well. Refrigerate until firm. Roll into a ball and roll over chopped pecans. Wrap with waxed paper and refrigerate until serving time. Serve with assorted crackers.

Nancy Olson
Clarksdale

BROTHER'S SHRIMP DIP

YIELD: 5 CUPS

1 pound fresh shrimp	1 to 2 teaspoons
½ cup horseradish	Worcestershire sauce
1 cup mayonnaise	¼ teaspoon cayenne pepper
8 ounces cream cheese, softened	

Boil and devein shrimp. Cut into bite-size pieces. Add remaining ingredients and mix well. Serve with melba rounds.

Tuck Reaves
Grenada, MS

Omit horseradish and mayonnaise. Substitute 8 ounces sour cream and ½ cup each of chopped celery and chopped onion.

Pam Mitchell
Lula

PARTY SHRIMP

SERVES: 6

4 tablespoons vinegar	2 large onions sliced thin
4 tablespoons prepared mustard	(use red onions)
	½ jar capers
2 teaspoons paprika	½ teaspoon salt
2 teaspoons celery seed	3 pounds peeled boiled
⅔ cup salad oil	shrimp

Mix above ingredients. Pour over 3 pounds peeled boiled shrimp. Let stand overnight. Serve with crackers.

Family Secret: Absolutely Divine!

Jo Ann White
Destin, Florida

CRABMEAT MOLD

YIELD: 4 CUPS

1 (10 ounce) can cream of
  mushroom soup
1 envelope unflavored
  gelatin
3 tablespoons cold water
¾ cup mayonnaise

1 (8 ounce) package cream
  cheese, softened
1 (6½ ounce) can crabmeat,
  drained
1 small onion, grated
1 cup finely chopped celery

Heat soup in a medium saucepan over low heat; remove from heat. Dissolve gelatin in cold water, add to soup, stirring well. Add remaining ingredients and spoon into an oiled 4 - cup mold. Chill until firm. Unmold and garnish with parsley. Serve with assorted crackers.

Sherry Eason
Mattson

FRIED SOYBEANS

My soybean farmer husband, Edwin, wanted me to find a way to fix soybeans for gifts. After many experiments and bushels of wasted soybeans, I came up with this tasty treat. Any farmer would be happy to give you some soybeans. If not, call Edwin!

SERVES: 4

4 cups raw soybeans
2 quarts water

Soybean oil, (cooking oil)
Salt

Wash soybeans and drain off any trash. Put soybeans in large mixing bowl with water (they will swell to about double). Soak at least four hours or overnight in the refrigerator. Drain all water off of soybeans. Use your deep fryer and cover the cooking area with newspaper as these splatter. Cook 1 cup at a time. When the soybeans start to float in the oil, and begin a popping sound, remove and drain on paper towels. This takes about 10 minutes. Sprinkle with salt while hot. Repeat until all beans are fried. These are a crunchy snack and will keep weeks in an airtight container.

Rosey B. Dulaney
Clarksdale

TOASTED PECANS

YIELD: 4 CUPS   OVEN: 375°

4 cups pecan halves   3 teaspoons salt
6 tablespoons margarine or
   butter

Melt margarine and pour over pecans. Sprinkle with salt, stir well.
Put pecans in shallow baking pan. Put pans in preheated oven, then
turn oven off. Let pecans stay in oven until cooled. Will not burn!

Roselyn Dulaney
Clarksdale

HEATON'S SUGAR ROASTED PECANS

YIELD: 4 CUPS   OVEN: 250°

4 cup pecan halves   1 teaspoon salt
3 tablespoons butter, melted   1 to 2 tablespoons sugar

Put pecans in a roasting pan 1-2 layers deep. Roast 30 minutes
stirring once. Remove from oven. Pour butter over pecans and stir
with wooden spoon until each pecan is coated. Return to oven for
30-40 minutes, stirring 3-4 times. Remove, add salt and sugar,
stirring to coat nuts and roast 5-10 minutes more. Store in airtight
container.

Mrs. Cliff Heaton
Lyon

Health Secret: Keep nutrient - rich foods on hand for snacks as
well as regular meals - fresh fruits, sliced raw vegetables, whole
grain muffins. A blend of unsweetened fruit juice and club soda
is a great alternative to soft drinks.

CRESCENT CHEESE SURPRISE

SERVES: 8 TO 10   OVEN: 350°

1 can crescent dinner rolls   1 (5 ounce) Havarti cheese
2 tablespoons dill and lemon
  seasoning

Roll out half of crescent rolls and make seams go together so it forms a rectangle. Sprinkle lemon and dill seasoning all over crescent rolls. Place cheese half on top of dough. Wrap dough around cheese like a present. Cut off excess dough and cut a bow for decorations on top. Bake 20 minutes or until brown.

Family Secret: This is attractive served with grapes that have been soaked in lemon juice then coated with fine sugar and placed on green leaves.

Chris B. Heaton
Clarksdale

CREAM CHEESE/CINNAMON BITS

YIELD: 2 DOZEN   OVEN: 350°

1 (8 ounce) cream cheese,   1 cup sugar
  softened   1 stick melted butter
1 egg yolk   4 tablespoons cinnamon
¼ cup sugar
8 slices thin white sandwich
  bread

Mix first three ingredients. Spread on bread which has had crusts removed and been flattened with a rolling pin. Roll up jelly roll style. Mix sugar and cinnamon. Dip each roll in melted butter, then in sugar and cinnamon. Bake fifteen minutes. Cut into thirds before serving. These can be frozen at this point and reheated in a microwave.

Linda Langston
Starkville

HOT CHEESE LOAF

SERVES: 8 TO 10   OVEN: 325°

1 large round loaf of
   Hawaiian bread
2 cups grated sharp Cheddar
   cheese
1½ cups of sour cream
1 bunch of green onions,
   chopped
1 tablespoon Worcestershire
   sauce

1 small jar dried beef,
   chopped
1 (4 ounce) can diced green
   chili peppers
1 (2 ounce) jar pimento,
   drained

Slice top off loaf and remove bread from center. Combine all ingredients and fill hollowed loaf. Put top slice on loaf and wrap in foil. Bake 1½ hours. Serve with corn chips.

Margaret Keeler
Clarksdale

FRIED CHEESE BALLS

We call these fried cheese balls "church puppies," a name they were given by a parishioner when they were served at a St. George's Episcopal Church Lenten luncheon.

YIELD: 14 TO 16 BALLS

2 cups grated American
   cheese
2 teaspoons flour

2 egg whites, beaten stiff
Cracker crumbs

Sprinkle flour over grated cheese. Mix cheese lightly with egg whites. Make into walnut-size balls. Roll in cracker crumbs. Fry in deep fat until brown.

Mary M. Thompson
Clarksdale

HOT BUTTERED BRIE

SERVES: 4 TO 6

½ cup butter
1 (4½ ounce) package Brie

1 (2¼ ounce) package sliced almonds

Melt butter in small skillet over medium heat. Add cheese round, turning cheese until it is slightly brown on both sides. Remove cheese to platter. Add almonds to butter and continue stirring until lightly browned. Remove almonds with slotted spoon and place on top of cheese. A little of the butter may be poured over all before serving.

Family Secret: Serve while warm with wheat crackers. Camembert is also good prepared this way.

Mrs. Lynn Kittle
Clarksdale

SHRIMP BITES IN PUFF PASTRY

OVEN: 400°

¼ cup minced green pepper
2 tablespoons minced onion
2 tablespoons margarine
2 tablespoons all-purpose flour
1 cup half-and-half cream
2 tablespoons dry sherry

1 can (4½ ounce) tiny shrimp, drained
1 tablespoon finely chopped pimento
¼ tablespoon salt
1 package puff pastry sheets
Eggs

Sauté pepper and onion in margarine until tender. Stir in flour and cook one minute longer, stirring constantly. Remove from heat and gradually blend in cream and sherry. Return to heat and cook, stirring constantly, until mixture comes to a boil. Remove from heat and stir in shrimp, pimiento, and salt. Set aside to cool completely. Thaw pastry sheets twenty minutes and unfold. Roll each sheet on floured surface to 12 inch square. Cut each sheet into 16-inch squares. Top each square with shrimp mixture. Brush edges with egg and fold in half to form triangle. Press edges together with fork tines. Brush with more egg. Cook on ungreased baking sheet for 10 to 12 minutes.

Mrs. Mary M. Thompson
Clarksdale

MUSHROOMS STUFFED WITH CRAB MEAT

SERVES: 8   OVEN: 400°

24 large fresh mushrooms
12 green onions, chopped
4 sprigs parsley, chopped
5 tablespoons margarine
¾ teaspoons Worcestershire
Salt and pepper to taste

1 tablespoon flour
½ cup cooking sherry or
  white wine
2 (7½ ounce) cans crab meat
1 pound sharp Cheddar
  cheese, grated

Wash mushrooms gently under running water and drain in colander. Trim stems; then cut off stems and chop along with onions and parsley. Sauté mushroom stems, onions and parsley in margarine in small skillet, adding Worcestershire, salt and pepper, for about 10 minutes. Stir in flour and then wine. Add crab meat last. Put caps in large shallow pan and salt lightly. Use teaspoon to divide mixture among mushrooms. Top with grated cheese and bake for 10 minutes, or until cheese is melted. Excellent as an appetizer, entree for luncheon or garnish for fillet of beef!

Gay Flowers
Mattson

CHESAPEAKE HOT MUSHROOM DIP

SERVES: 4 TO 6   OVEN: 350°

1 (8 ounce) can of mushroom
  pieces and stems (drained)
¾ cup of mayonnaise
1 cup of shredded Cheddar
  cheese

⅓ cup Parmesan cheese
½ package dry herb salad
  dressing mix

Drain mushrooms and chop in food processor. Mix with all the rest of ingredients and stir. Bake in small ovenproof bowls. Sprinkle top with extra Cheddar and Parmesan cheeses. Bake twenty minutes and serve with wheat crackers.

Betty Hood
Gunnison

HOT CRABMEAT PIE

SERVES: 10   OVEN: 350°

1 pound of lump crabmeat
1 tablespoon of horseradish
1 teaspoon of grated lemon
  rind
½ teaspoon of monosodium
  glutamate

Dash of hot sauce
2 cups of mayonnaise
¾ cup of grated sharp
  Cheddar cheese

Mix together all ingredients except cheese. Add other seasonings, if you like (grated onion, Worcestershire, garlic). Put ingredients in a 10 - inch pyrex pie plate. Spread evenly and cover with cheese. Heat about 20-25 minutes or until mixture bubbles. Run under broiler for a few minutes until cheese is lightly brown. Place pie plate in center of tray and encircle with crackers.

Family Secret: This is so good and very simple to make.

Gay Flowers
Clarksdale

HOT CRABMEAT

SERVES: 15 AS APPETIZER, 8 AS ENTRÉE   OVEN: 350°

4 tablespoons butter
4 tablespoons flour
2 cups half and half cream,
  room temperature
3 green onions, chopped
1 teaspoon lemon juice

1 teaspoon parsley
Salt, pepper, cayenne pepper
  to taste
1 teaspoon Worcestershire
  sauce
1 pound lump crabmeat

Prepare a cream sauce in double boiler. Melt butter, add flour and blend. Slowly stir in half and half cream, cooking until thick. Add all other seasonings. Pick crabmeat from shells and add to mixture. Serve from chafing dish with melba rounds or pastry cups. Also can be placed in ramekins, topped with buttered bread crumbs and baked for 15 minutes or until bubbly hot.

Jane Longino
Clarksdale

SUMMER SAUSAGE

YIELD: 5 TO 6 ROLLS   OVEN: 200°

5 pounds ground chuck
7½ teaspoons Tender Quick
  Salt
4½ teaspoons garlic salt

4½ teaspoons coarse ground
  black pepper (or pepper-
  corns)
8 to 10 drops liquid smoke

Mix ingredients together (with hands) in large bowl. Shape into rolls (about 5 to 6 depending on the size you make them) and wrap in plastic wrap. Refrigerate 24 to 36 hours; the rolls will form their own casing. Take wrapping off and bake 4 hours. Cool and enjoy!

Family Secret: This is good with cheese, crackers, and a tangy mustard.

Marilyn Young
Clarksdale

PITA B'S

OVEN: 250°

1 package pita bread rounds
Butter
Dill weed

Seasoned salt
Parmesan cheese (grated)

Butter pita bread after cutting into small wedges. Sprinkle well with seasoned salt and dill weed, then with Parmesan cheese. Place on ungreased cookie sheet and bake until slightly browned, usually about 30 to 45 minutes. Allow to cool before storing in tins.

Lynn Kittle
Clarksdale

Health Secret: A great sour cream substitute is a blend of low fat cottage cheese with 1 to 2 tablespoons of yogurt.

STUFFED ARTICHOKES

SERVES: 4-6   OVEN: 350°

1 cup cracker crumbs
1 cup seasoned bread crumbs
2 cups Parmesan cheese
2 bunches green onions with
  tops, chopped fine

½ cup grated Cheddar cheese
Olive oil
4 to 6 artichokes

Mix first 5 ingredients together. Add olive oil a little at a time until mixture sticks together. Cut points from artichoke leaves. Put stuffing in between leaves. Place in shallow baking dish with about ½ inch of water in bottom. Dot each artichoke with butter. Bake covered for 2 hours, or until tender. Add more water, if needed.

Evelyn Demilio
Clarksdale

DEVILED HAM PUFFS

YIELD: 24   OVEN: 350°

1 (8 ounce) package cream
  cheese, softened
1 egg yolk, beaten
1 teaspoon onion juice
½ teaspoon baking powder
Salt to taste

¼ teaspoon horseradish
¼ teaspoon red hot sauce
24 small bread rounds
2 (2¼ ounce) cans deviled
  ham

Blend together the cheese, egg yolk, onion juice, baking powder, salt, horseradish, and hot sauce. Add deviled ham and mix. Toast small bread round on one side. Spread untoasted side with deviled ham mixture and bake for 10 to 12 minutes until puffed and brown. Serve hot.

Susan Connell
Clarksdale

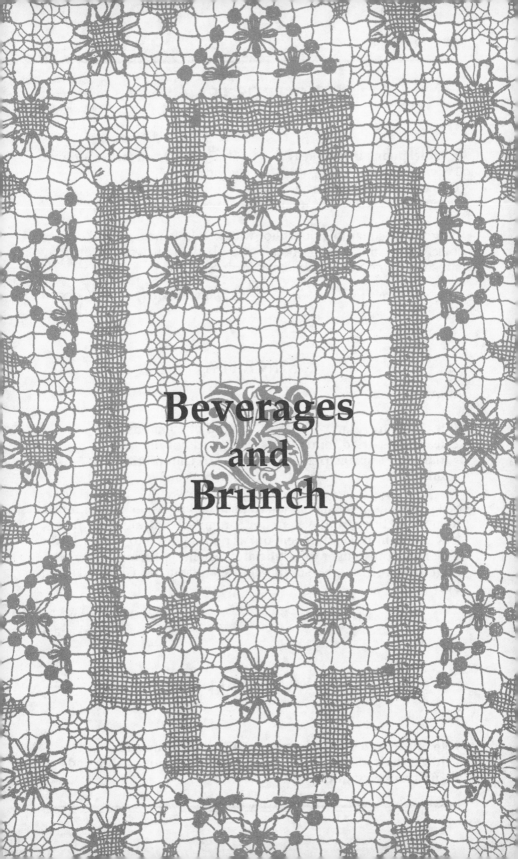

Beverages
and
Brunch

CITRUS TEA

YIELD: 1 GALLON

4 tablespoons instant tea   1 (6 ounce) can frozen orange
1½ cups sugar   juice
1 (6 ounce) can frozen
   lemonade

Put tea and sugar in 1 quart hot water. Add lemonade and orange juice. Place in 1 gallon container and fill with water. You may substitute 2 family size tea bags for instant tea.

Maggie Tyner, Susan Connell
Clarksdale

MINT TEA

SERVES: 8

5 tea bags (regular)   Rind of 2 lemons
2 teaspoons dried mint   8 cups boiling water
   flakes or 5 sprigs fresh   ½ cup lemon juice
   mint   1½ cups sugar

Steep tea bags, mint and lemon rinds in boiling water for 5 minutes. Remove all three from water after 5 minutes. (if using dried flakes, leave them in and strain them out as pouring tea into pitcher.) Add lemon juice and sugar (or artificial sweetener), stirring as you add. Pour mixture through a strainer into a large pitcher. Chill and serve over ice.

Mrs. Lee Graves, Jr.
Clarksdale

ORANGE BLUSH

YIELD: 6

1 (6 ounce) can frozen orange   4 tablespoons sugar
   juice, thawed   1 pint (16 ounce) club soda
1 cup cranberry juice

CONTINUED, ORANGE BLUSH

Combine undiluted orange juice, cranberry juice, and sugar: Chill thoroughly. Just before serving, stir in the club soda and pour over ice.

Family Secret: This may be prepared ahead except for the addition of the club soda.

Mary M. Thompson
Clarksdale

ORANGE SUNSHINE

YIELD: 4 SMALL GLASSES

1 small can orange juice, slightly thawed
1 cup milk

½ cup sugar
Ice

Mix first three ingredients in blender. Fill blender with ice and mix on highest speed until smooth.

Family Secret: A special treat when you have guests for breakfast.

Dottie Seymore
Tutwiler

ALICE LEE'S BLOODY MARY

YIELD: 1 GALLON

48 ounces tomato juice
48 ounces vegetable juice
2 to 3 teaspoons horseradish
½ cup lemon juice
5 tablespoons Worchester-
shire sauce

1 teaspoon salt
2 to 3 drops hot sauce
2 cups vodka

Mix all ingredients chill and serve with celery sticks.

Alice Lee Hayes
Clarksdale

COFFEE PUNCH

SERVES: 100

1 gallon extra strong coffee, cooled (16) cups
2 quarts milk
1 quart of half and half cream
1 cup sugar
4 teaspoons vanilla
1 gallon coffee ice cream
1 gallon vanilla ice cream
1 pint whipped cream

Mix the first three ingredients. Add sugar and vanilla to taste. Pour over ice cream and "dab" whipped cream on top.

FOR SMALLER GROUPS:

SERVES:10

1 pint milk
2 quarts strong coffee, cooled
2 teaspoons vanilla
½ cup sugar
1 quart vanilla ice cream
½ pint whipping cream
grated nutmeg

Susan Connell
Clarksdale

EGG NOG

YIELD: 3 QUARTS

16 egg yolks
12 tablespoons sugar
1 fifth of bourbon
1 quart whipping cream, stiffly whipped (no egg whites)

Beat yolks until light in color and stiff. Add sugar 1 tablespoon at a time beating slowly, then slowly add bourbon 1 tablespoon at a time. Fold in stiffly whipped cream.

Jewell Graeber
Marks

BEIGNETS

SERVES: 8 TO 10

½ cup butter
1 cup water
2 tablespoons sugar
1 cup flour

2 eggs, plus 1 egg yolk
Oil
Confectioners sugar

In a heavy bottomed pan boil first three ingredients. Add flour all at once, stirring vigorously over heat until mixture leaves sides of pan. Remove from heat. Add eggs one at a time, beating well after each addition. Drop egg size spoonfuls of mixture into 375° oil and fry until brown. Shake in bag of confectioners sugar to coat.

Sherry Donald
Clarksdale

BREAKFAST PIZZA

SERVES: 8   OVEN: 375°

1 pound bulk pork sausage
1 (8 ounce) package
   refrigerated crescent rolls
1 cup frozen loose-packed
   hash browns
1 cup sharp Cheddar cheese

5 eggs
¼ cup milk
½ teaspoon salt
⅛ teaspoon pepper
2 tablespoons grated
   Parmesan cheese

Cook sausage in skillet until browned. Drain excess fat. Separate crescent dough into eight triangles. Place in ungreased 12 inch pizza pan with points toward center. Press over bottom and up sides to form a crust. Seal perforations. Spoon sausage over crust. Sprinkle with thawed potatoes. Top with Cheddar cheese. In a bowl, beat together eggs, milk, salt, and pepper. Pour into crust. Sprinkle with Parmesan. Bake for 25 to 30 minutes.

Eileen M. Casburn
Sumner

Health Secret: Jazzing up fiber - Add 1 to 2 tablespoons sunflower seeds, pecans, pinenuts or raisins and dates to cereal. Or toast oatmeal and pinenuts and add to vanilla low - fat yogurt.

FARMERS BREAKFAST

SERVES: 6 TO 8   OVEN: 350°

6 medium potatoes   1 dozen eggs
1 pound bacon   Salt and pepper to taste
2 large onions, sliced thin

Cook potatoes until almost done. Peel and slice. Snip bacon and fry
until almost crisp. Drain. Add sliced onions and sauté. In a 9 x 12
inch pan, put a layer of potatoes, then layer of onions and bacon
until both are gone. Beat eggs. Add salt and pepper. Pour over top
of vegetable layers. Bake uncovered for 40 minutes.

Emily Cooper
Clarksdale

GERMAN EGG PANCAKES

*My father-in-law, August Surholt, Sr., came from Germany to
the Mississippi Delta in 1921 driving the first International
cotton picker to our community. Fred's fondest memories of his
father were the many German meals he prepared. These German
Egg Pancakes were always a treat on mornings they rose early
to go hunting or fishing together.*

YIELD: 6 PANCAKES 9 INCHES IN SIZE

4 eggs   1 teaspoon vanilla
Pinch of salt   1 cup plain flour
2 tablespoons sugar   1 cup milk

Mix all ingredients in blender. Add more milk, if necessary, until
thin pancake consistency. Pour mixture in consistent circle forming
a spiral into ½ inch hot grease on stove top. Turn when brown on
one side. Drain on paper towel. Similar to a funnel cake.

Family Secret: Serve with baby link sausages and syrup.

Donna Surholt (Mrs. Fred Surholt)
Clarksdale

CHEESE SOUFFLÉ

SERVES: 6   OVEN: 350°

4 thick slices of bread   2 cups milk
2 cups grated, aged Cheddar   Salt
   cheese   White pepper
3 eggs   Dash of hot sauce (several)

Remove edges from bread. Cut into cubes and place in layers with cheese in baking dish. Beat whole eggs until light. Add milk and seasonings and pour over bread. Let it stand 30 minutes or longer. Bake 40 minutes

Georgia Salmon Antici
Clarksdale

SOUFFLÉ OF GRITS

SERVES: 8   OVEN: 350°

4 cups boiling water   4 tablespoons flour
1 cup grits, uncooked   1 tablespoon dry mustard
1 teaspoon salt   4 cups sharp Cheddar cheese,
½ cup butter or margarine   separated
4 eggs, separated

Add grits and salt to boiling water. Stir in butter; cook according to package directions. Pour cooked grits into large mixing bowl and beat in egg yolks, one at a time. Sift flour over grits. Add mustard and 3 cups cheese. Mix well. Whip egg whites. Fold into grits. Pour into greased 8 inch casserole. Bake 45 minutes.

Family Secret: This can be made the day before and baked just before you are ready to serve it. It is wonderful served with doves, broiled tomatoes, hot biscuits, home-made preserves, and plenty of coffee.

Mrs. Gus Brown, Jr.
Marks

HAM AND CHEESE QUICHE

SERVES: 4 TO 6   OVEN: 350°

1 large onion, chopped
¼ cup margarine
1 can (10¾ ounce) can cream
  of chicken or celery soup
4 eggs
½ cup cream

1 cup cheese (Cheddar),
  shredded
1 large deep dish frozen pie
  crust
¼ cup bacon bits
¾ cup diced ham

Sauté onion in microwave with margarine until tender. While the onion is sautéing, mix soup with eggs and cream. Sprinkle the bottom of pie crust generously with ham and bacon bits. Slowly mix soup mixture with onion until well blended. Fold in cheese. Pour into pie crust and bake around 45 minutes (will be lightly brown and firm in the middle when done.)

Kathy Davis
Clarksdale

SHRIMP AND CRAB QUICHE

SERVES: 6   OVEN: 350°

1 (7½ ounce) can shrimp
  (wash and drain)
1 (7½ ounce) can crabmeat
  (wash and drain)
⅓ cup chopped green onion
8 ounces Swiss cheese,
  grated
2 tablespoons flour

1 deep-dish pie crust, unbaked
2 eggs
½ cup milk
1 cup mayonnaise (regular)
Dash salt, pepper and garlic
  powder

Place first 5 ingredients in plastic bag. Shake to coat shrimp and crab with flour. Then put into pie crust. Mix next 3 ingredients and seasonings. Beat with wire whisk and pour over shrimp mixture in pie shell. Bake for 1 hours.

Family Secret: Serve with fresh fruit or green salad.

Betty Hood
Gunnison

GRANOLA

YIELD: 9 TO 10 CUPS   OVEN: 325°

6 cups old-fashioned rolled
  oats, uncooked
1 cup shredded coconut
1 cup wheat germ
½ cup sesame seeds
1 cup coarsely chopped
  pecans
¼ cup vegetable oil (not olive
  oil)

½ cup honey
¾ teaspoon salt
1½ teaspoons vanilla
⅓ cup water
⅓ cup brown sugar
1 cup raisins

Mix first five ingredients in large container. Mix remaining ingredients. except raisins, in a small bowl. Pour liquid mixture over dry mixture. Toss to coat evenly. Spread onto two 11 inch by 17 inch greased cookie sheets. Bake for 35 to 40 minutes, turning mixture with a spatula once. Be careful not to burn. When mixture is cooled thoroughly, add 1 cup raisins. Mix. Store in tight container.

Family Secret: Lower in fat and sugar than most commercial granolas. It is great added to non-fat yogurt with your favorite fruit.

Emily Cooper
Clarksdale

WAFFLES

YIELD: 6 TO 8

2 cups flour
2 tablespoons sugar
1 teaspoon salt
3 teaspoons baking powder

2 eggs, separated
1¾ cups milk
4 tablespoons melted butter

Sift dry ingredients together in mixing bowl. Add egg yolks and milk, slowly beating until batter is smooth. Add melted butter and fold in stiffly beaten egg whites. Cook on waffle iron.

Family Secret: Before folding in egg whites, you can add 1 cup blueberries, drained pineapple, or chopped nuts.

Mrs. Lee Graves, Sr.
Clarksdale

JOHNNY APPLESEED FRENCH TOAST

SERVES: 4

1 can (21 ounce) apple pie
  filling
1 tablespoon brown sugar
1 teaspoon cinnamon
4 eggs

½ cup milk
¼ teaspoon salt
4 slices bread
2 tablespoons butter

Empty pie filling into saucepan. Stir in sugar and cinnamon. Warm over low heat. Beat eggs in pie plate. Mix in milk and salt. Put butter on heated griddle and cover surface. Soak both sides of each slice of bread in egg mixture for 10 to 15 seconds. Cook on griddle until nicely browned on both sides. To serve: put each piece of French toast on a plate and spoon about ½ cup of the hot apple pie filling over. (Refrigerate leftover pie filling to use another day).

Family Secret: For an extra special treat, put a scoop of vanilla ice cream on top of each apple-covered French toast slice.

Nelda Mooney
Friars Point

Health Secret: Children can decide how much they want to eat, but adults should set the healthy and balanced dietary patterns for their children to follow.

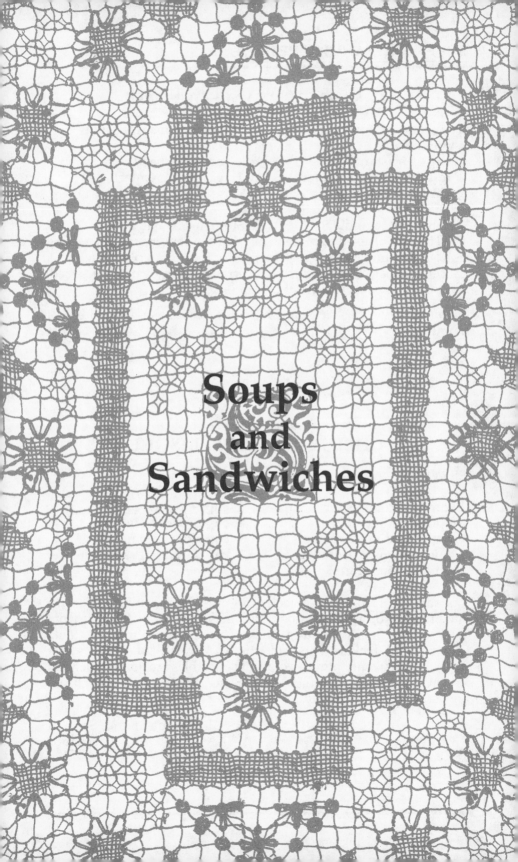

Soups
and
Sandwiches

INSTANT CREAM SOUP MIX

2 cups non-fat dry milk
  powder
¾ cups cornstarch
2 to 4 tablespoons instant
  chicken bouillon

2 tablespoons dry onion
  flakes
1 teaspoon basil
1 teaspoon pepper

Combine all ingredients. Mix well. Store in a container with a tight lid. This can be used in place of one can condensed soup by mixing as follows: mix ⅓ cup dry mix with 1¼ cups cold water in a saucepan. Cook over medium heat, stirring constantly until thickened. Add to a recipe as you would a can of soup.

Family Secret: This does not have the sodium or fat content of canned soups.

Emily Cooper
Clarksdale

CHEESY BROCCOLI BISQUE

SERVES: 6

1 cup sliced leeks (or ¼ cup
  spring onion)
1 cup sliced mushrooms
3 tablespoons margarine
3 tablespoons flour

3 cups chicken broth
1 cup broccoli florets
1 cup light cream
1 cup shredded sharp cheese

In a large saucepan sauté leeks and mushrooms until tender. Do not brown. Add flour and cook, stirring until bubbly. Remove from heat and gradually blend in chicken broth. Return to heat. Cook, stirring until thickened and smooth. Add broccoli and reduce heat and simmer twenty minutes or until vegetables are tender. Blend in cream and cheese. Simmer until heated thoroughly and cheese melts. Serve immediately.

Mrs. John Homes Sherard
Sherard

BROCCOLI SOUP

SERVES: 12

5 or 6 pieces chicken, legs
  and thighs
Stock from chicken
2 pints hot water
2 large onions, thinly sliced
3 ribs celery, thinly sliced
2 large cloves garlic, minced
3 chicken bouillon cubes

2 (10 ounce) packages frozen
  broccoli spears, thawed
  (fresh broccoli may be
  used)
1 cup vermicelli or tiny soup
  noodles (break vermicelli 3
  to 4 times)
Salt and pepper to taste

Boil chicken pieces until cooked, then debone. Strain stock and reserve. Start 2 pints water to boil in heavy pot with onions, celery, garlic, and bouillon cubes and strained stock from chicken. Cook until onions and celery are transparent. As water boils down, add hot water to pot; add cooked chicken and let cook on medium-low to simmer 15 to 30 minutes. Chop broccoli stems into ¼ inch pieces and let cook about 15 minutes. Add broccoli flowerets in bite-size pieces and cook until tender (about 10 minutes). Add pasta and cook until it is al dente. Season with salt and pepper to taste. If soup gets too thick, just add hot water.

Family Secret: Left over chicken may be used.

Carolyn Stringer
Clarksdale

COLD CUCUMBER-AVOCADO SOUP

SERVES: 4

1 cup peeled cucumbers
½ avocado, ripe
2 green onions and tops,
  chopped

1 cup chicken broth
1 cup sour cream
2 tablespoons lemon juice
Salt, pepper

Put all the ingredients in food processor. Blend. Pour in container and chill.

Family Secret: Wonderful for a summer luncheon.

Jane Longino
Clarksdale

CUCUMBER AND SPINACH SOUP

SERVES: 6

Salt and pepper to taste
1 onion, chopped
1 large potato, chopped
1 leek, chopped
3 sprigs fresh parsley, chopped
2 cubes chicken base
1½ pints of water
½ bunch blanched spinach, chopped

2 peeled cucumbers, chopped
½ cup sour cream
1 tablespoon mayonnaise
1 teaspoon horseradish
Juice of 2 lemons
Drops of hot sauce
1 avocado, chopped

Combine first 5 ingredients in a large saucepan with water. Boil 20 minutes. Cool. Blend in food processor or blender with two on-off pulses. Mixture should have very small pieces. Blend spinach and cucumbers in same manner. Add to first mixture. Add remaining ingredients and blend well. Add the avocado just before serving.

Patsy Maclin
Clarksdale

RISI SPINACI (SPINACH WITH RICE SOUP)

SERVES: 4 TO 6

1 (12 ounce) cans of chicken broth
1 (10 ounce) package of frozen chopped spinach
1½ cups cooked rice

3 tablespoons tomato paste
Parmesan cheese (to sprinkle on top of individual servings)

Defrost spinach in microwave. Add to chicken broth. Heat through on top of stove. Add rice and tomato paste and continue heating until hot. Sprinkle each serving with Parmesan cheese.

Family Secret: Can be used as an appetizer or as a meal by itself. More rice can be used if thicker soup is desired. Also if you want to cook the raw rice in the soup, add an extra can of chicken broth.

Toni Malvezzi Hardin
Duncan

BAKED ONION SOUP

SERVES: 6 TO 8

5 cups or about 3 large
  yellow onions
2 tablespoons vegetable oil
½ teaspoon salt
¼ teaspoon sugar
3 tablespoons flour

5 cups canned beef broth
3 cups water
½ cup dry white wine
Salt and pepper to taste
1½ cups Swiss cheese, grated

Slice onions thinly. Cook slowly in oil in covered, heavy 4 quart saucepan for 15 minutes. Uncover, stir in salt and sugar and raise heat to medium. Cook, stirring frequently, for about 30 minutes, until onions are a golden brown. Sprinkle in flour and stir for 2 to 3 minutes. Warm beef broth, water, and wine in another pan. Stir into onion mixture. Simmer, partly covered, for 2 to 3 hours. Add salt and pepper to taste. To make bread topping, place bread slices in single layer on cookie sheet and bake for 30 minutes at 325°. Pour soup into individual oven proof soup pots. Float toast rounds on top of soup. Sprinkle with grated cheese. Bake at 325° for 20 minutes.

Family Secret: Serve with toasted bread rounds and salad.

Emily Cooper
Clarksdale

POTATO SOUP

SERVES: 6 TO 8

¼ cup margarine
4 cups potatoes, diced
1 cup finely chopped celery
1 medium onion, chopped

4 cups chicken broth
1 (8 ounce) container sour
  cream (optional)
Salt and pepper to taste

In a a large saucepan, melt margarine and sauté potatoes, celery and onions. Add broth and simmer until vegetables are tender. A dollop of sour cream may be added to each bowl as it is served.

Family Secret: For a creamy soup, add a 13 ounce can evaporated milk.

Sherry Donald
Clarksdale

BEEF VEGETABLE SOUP

SERVES: 12

1½ pounds stew meat
4 tablespoons oil
1 onion, chopped
1 stalk celery, chopped
8 cups water
2 (15 ounce) cans of tomato
  sauce
1 beef bouillon cube
3 carrots, peeled and
  chopped

6 potatoes, chopped
1 (8 ounce) can corn
1 (8 ounce) can cut green
  beans
1 (8 ounce) can of peas
1 teaspoon garlic powder
Salt and pepper to taste

In a a 10 to 12 gallon cooking pot, add oil and brown stew meat, chopped onions and celery. After browned, add tomato sauce, water, bouillon cube, chopped carrots and potatoes. Bring to boil and stir. Turn down heat to low and cook about an hour, then add remaining ingredients. Heat through.

Meg Agostinelli
Lyon

CHEESY VEGETABLE SOUP

SERVES: 10 TO 12

1½ to 2 cups diced potatoes
1½ to 2 cups chopped green
  onions
1½ to 2 cups chopped celery
1½ to 2 cups carrots
6 tablespoons margarine
6 cups chicken broth,
  divided

1 cup flour
4 cups milk
1 (16 ounce) jar pasteurized
  processed cheese spread
2 tablespoons prepared
  mustard

Boil carrots, and potatoes for 15 minutes in 2 cups of chicken broth in 5 to 6 quart pot. Sauté onion and celery in margarine. Stir 1 cup flour into onion mixture until smooth. Stir in 2 cups of broth. Combine onion-celery mixture, the remaining 2 cups broth and milk with the carrots and potatoes. Add processed cheese spread and 2 tablespoons prepared mustard. Heat well but do not boil.

Barbara Agostinelli and Marie Stonestreet
Clarksdale

MEXICAN CHEESE SOUP

SERVES: 4

1 tablespoon margarine
½ cup onion, finely chopped
½ cup celery, finely chopped
1 (14½ ounce) can chicken
  broth·
¾ cup pasteurized processed
  cheese
2 tablespoons sour cream

⅓ cup mild salsa sauce
2 cups of milk
8 to 10 drops of hot sauce
3 tablespoons green pepper,
  finely chopped
1 tablespoon fresh chives,
  diced

In a large saucepan, melt margarine. Add the celery and onion and sauté over low heat until the vegetables are softened. Add the chicken broth and simmer. Cut cheese into small cubes. Add to broth. Cook over low heat, stirring occasionally, until cheese is melted. Stir in sour cream, salsa, milk and hot sauce and continue cooking over low heat until thoroughly heated. Be careful not to boil. Add the green pepper and heat 2 to 3 more minutes. Put in soup cups and sprinkle with chives. Serve with tortilla chips.

Sarah Miles
Clarksdale

MULLIGATAWNY SOUP

If you want your guests to rave, make this Indian creation full of subtle flavors, which became a favorite American dish a century ago.

SERVES: 8

2 tablespoons butter
½ cup onion, minced
1 small clove garlic, crushed
2 tablespoons flour
1 tablespoon curry powder
1 quart chicken stock

1 pint half-and-half
1 raw apple, peeled and
  chopped fine
1 tablespoon salt
Dash of pepper

Melt the butter in the pot you are going to make the soup in. Add onion and crushed garlic and cook over low heat until the onion is soft. Add the flour and curry powder and cook 2 minutes. Add chicken stock, stirring constantly. Salt and pepper. Then add half-and-half stirring well. Add the apple last, 10 minutes before serving.

Mrs. W. J. Brady
Clarksdale

EGG DROP SOUP

SERVES: 5

5 cups chicken broth
1 cup frozen peas
½ cup diced canned mush-
  rooms
¼ cup diced uncooked
  chicken

1 teaspoon soy sauce
Cornstarch mixture (2 tablespoons cornstarch mixed
  with 2 tablespoons water)
2 eggs (beaten)
A few drops of sesame oil

In a covered soup pot, place chicken broth. Bring to a boil. Add peas, mushrooms, chicken, and soy sauce. Stir in cornstarch mixture. Bring to a boil. Lower the heat. Stir in eggs until eggs separate in shreds. Season to taste with salt. Add sesame oil.

Sally Chow
Clarksdale

GATES GOURMET GUMBO

SERVES: 10

4 Mallard ducks
3 quarts water (or more)
1½ sticks margarine
1 cup flour
1 small stalk celery, chopped
3 cloves garlic, minced
3 to 4 medium onions,
  chopped
1 large bell pepper chopped
1 bunch green onions,
  chopped
1 can tomato paste
2 teaspoons monosodium
  glutamate

1 teaspoon oregano
2 tablespoons salt
1½ to 2 tablespoons fresh
  gumbo filé*
2 (20 ounce) cans tomatoes
2 tablespoons dry parsley
1 teaspoon thyme
1 tablespoon black pepper
½ teaspoon red pepper
1 (10 ounce) package frozen
  cut okra (optional)

CONTINUED, GATES GOURMET GUMBO

Place ducks in stewing pot with water and cook until tender; debone. In a skillet, melt margarine, blend in flour and brown slowly to make a roux (gravy). Strain two quarts of broth from the pan the ducks were cooked in, add roux, and mix well. Add all the other ingredients in a large pot with duck meat and broth, and simmer approximately three hours, stirring often.

Family Secret: Serve over a mound of long grain and wild rice mixture with hot corn bread sticks on the side. *Use gumbo filé that you have just purchased. It loses its flavor during storage.

Alex B. Gates
Sumner

HUNGARIAN PAPRIKASH

SERVES: 10

1 large hen (4 pounds)	2 heaping tablespoons
4 to 5 chopped onions (large	cornstarch
pieces)	2 (8 ounce) cartons sour
2 to 4 tablespoons cooking oil	cream
(as needed)	1 (12 ounce) package egg
2 to 4 tablespoons paprika	noodles

Boil hen in plenty of water with salt and pepper until done. Remove meat from bone; cut into large pieces. Reserve liquid. Sauté onions in large container in oil until tender. Stir in paprika. Add chicken stock and let come to boil. Add two heaping tablespoons cornstarch to sour cream, mixing well. Pour some of the chicken broth into cream until it is of pouring consistency. Pour this into broth stirring constantly to keep from curdling. Let cook about thirty minutes. Add noodles that have been cooked and drained. Add boned chicken.

Georgia Abraham Wilson
Clarksdale

POLISH SAUSAGE SOUP

SERVES: 8

2 tablespoons butter
½ cup chopped onion
½ cup chopped celery
1 pound polish sausage, cut
  in pieces
1 (10¾ ounce) can consommé
½ can water

2 tablespoons vinegar
½ teaspoon thyme
1 small head cabbage,
  shredded
1 (4 ounce) can mushrooms
2 to 3 medium potatoes,
  diced

Sauté sausage, onion, and celery in butter. Add one can consommé and water. Season with vinegar, salt to taste, thyme, shredded cabbage and sliced mushrooms. Cook about 30 minutes. Add potatoes and cook 30 to 45 minutes more until potatoes are done. Very good and different.

Judy B. Carlson
Clarksdale

BRUNSWICK STEW

YIELD: 5 GALLONS

10 pounds deboned squirrel
  meat (20 to 25 squirrels)
3 pounds deboned chicken
  meat (2 large hens)
2 pounds of ham
2 pounds of margarine
10 large chopped onions
4 (6 ounce) cans of tomato
  paste
3 pounds of frozen okra
4 (16 ounce) cans of whole,
  peeled tomatoes
7 pounds of diced potatoes
1 pound of diced carrots

4 (15 ounce) cans of lima
  beans, drained
3 (16 ounce) cans of cream
  style corn
3 (16 ounce) cans of whole
  corn, drained
1½ tablespoons thyme
2 tablespoons of black
  pepper
2 tablespoons of red pepper
1 tablespoon of salt
1 (10 ounce) bottle of
  Worcestershire sauce

CONTINUED, BRUNSWICK STEW

Cook squirrels and chickens until tender, debone and set aside until ready to add to the stew. Refrigerate if necessary. Strain and reserve broth. Melt margarine in pot, add chopped onions, and cook until onions are tender. Boil approximately 1 gallon of reserve broth in large pot, add diced carrots and cook for a few minutes. Than add diced potatoes and frozen okra and continue cooking until almost done but still slightly crunchy. Put carrots, potatoes, and okra into pot or roaster with onions, add broth in which vegetables were cooked and extra broth if necessary. Add tomato paste, tomatoes, black pepper, red pepper, thyme and salt. Cook over low heat until carrots and potatoes are tender. Stir gently but often to keep from sticking. Add broth as necessary. When potatoes and carrots are done, add lima beans, cream style corn, whole corn, Worcestershire sauce, and meat. STIR CONTINUOUSLY until stew bubbles lightly. Remove from heat and let cool, then correct seasoning.

Alex Gates
Sumner

NELL'S CHICKEN VELVET SOUP

Soon after we became neighbors, Nell Stribling Bobo brought me this wonderful chicken soup when I was ill with the flu.

SERVES: 15

⅔ cup butter
1½ cups flour
12 cups chicken stock
2 cups warm milk
2 cups warm cream

3 cups finely chopped chicken
1 teaspoon salt
1 teaspoon pepper

Melt butter, add flour and cook on low heat until well blended. Add 4 cups hot chicken stock, warm milk and cream. Cook slowly, stirring frequently until thick. Add remaining 8 cups chicken stock and the chicken and heat until boiling. Season with salt and pepper.

Eva Connell
Clarksdale

ITALIAN CHICKEN SOUP

YIELD: LOTS

5 to 6 pound hen
3 tablespoons Aline's Northern Italian seasoning

1 (8 ounce) can tomato sauce
½ teaspoon salt
½ teaspoon black pepper

Wash hen and put in very large soup pot. Cover with cold water about two inches above hen. Boil. Skim off foam as it appears. Add seasoning, tomato sauce, salt and pepper. Continue simmering, turning hen 2 to 3 times until hen is cooked, about 2 hours. Take out hen. Add rice noodles or anything you want in soup. Optional: Add 2 cups chopped hen.

ALINE'S NORTHERN ITALIAN SEASONING:

YIELD: 2 QUARTS

1 bunch parsley
1 whole stalk celery (6 to 7 pieces)

5 or 6 onions
10 individual cloves garlic

Wash each of these separately. Chop separately in food processor. Mix all together. You can put in jar and keep in refrigerator for months. Take out 2 to 3 tablespoons as needed. Or you can freeze in sandwich bags; keeps for a year. You can use this basic seasoning in soup, meatballs, meatloaf, top of turkey, chicken, etc.

Aline Alias
Clarksdale

"SOMETHING GOOD"

SERVES: 6 TO 8

Mix:
1 (13 ounce) can evaporated milk
1 (10½ ounce) can chicken gumbo

1 (10½ ounce) can pepper pot soup
1 (6 ounce) can crabmeat

Add a little hot sauce, if you want! Heat and serve!

Mrs. Leon Bramlett
Clarksdale

LOW-CAL CHICKEN SOUP

SERVES: 6 TO 8

4 whole boneless skinless
  chicken breasts
1 box lite lemon chicken dry
  soup mix (all 3 packages)
4 ounces English peas-no salt
1 onion, chopped
1 bell pepper, chopped
1 carrot, chopped
4 to 6 ounces mild thick and
  chunky taco salsa
1 (6 ounce) can vegetable
  juice
½ cup macaroni shells

Boil chicken in enough water to cover. Cool broth and skim off any fat. Cube chicken. Add all other ingredients to broth and simmer several hours.

Family Secret: A tasty low-cal soup.

Louella Graves
Clarksdale

OYSTER BISQUE

SERVES: 6

4 stalks celery, chopped
4 carrots, chopped
6 tablespoons margarine
2 tablespoons four
1 pint half-and-half
2 dozen oysters
2 cups milk
Parsley, salt, pepper and
  Worchestershire to taste

Chop and cook vegetables until tender in 2 tablespoons margarine. Make white sauce by melting 2 tablespoons margarine; add 2 tablespoons flour and mix well; add half-and-half and stir until thick. Add vegetables to sauce. Cook oysters until edges curl. Add to bisque. Add 2 cups milk and season with parsley, salt, pepper and Worchestershire sauce.

Margaret Sandifer
Clarksdale

CHICKEN AND SAUSAGE GUMBO

SERVES: 8

1 3 pound chicken, cut up
½ teaspoon salt
¼ teaspoon black pepper
1 pound smoked sausage
    (slice into bite-size pieces)
⅓ cup vegetable oil
½ cup flour
1 large onion, chopped
1 green pepper, chopped
2 ribs celery chopped
2 cloves garlic minced

2 cups hot chicken broth
1 quart hot water
Salt and pepper to taste
¾ cup cooked okra (optional)
1 pint oysters (optional)
¾ cup chopped green onion
    tops
¼ cup chopped parsley
Hot cooked rice
Filé (when okra is cooked,
    omit filé)

Season chicken with salt and pepper. Brown chicken and sausage in oil in heavy Dutch oven. Remove chicken from pan and reserve. Stir flour into drippings. Reduce heat to low; cook, stirring constantly to make a roux. Stir until roux is a caramel color. Add onions, green pepper, celery, and garlic to roux. Sauté 10 to 15 minutes, stirring occasionally. Add chicken, sausage, hot chicken broth, and hot water. Cold broth and water can cause roux to curdle. Add salt and pepper to taste. Heat to boiling; reduce heat and simmer 1½ hours or until chicken is tender. Add okra and oysters (if desired), parsley, and onion tops. Cover and cook 10 minutes. Remove from heat and let stand 10 minutes. Serve gumbo over rice. Filé powder may be sprinkled on by individuals (½ teaspoon per serving). Omit filé if okra was used.

Carolyn Stringer
Clarksdale

CRAB & SHRIMP GUMBO

SERVES: 8 TO 10

3 pound fryer, cut up
1 small stalk celery, chopped
2 medium bell peppers,
    chopped
4 large onions, chopped
6 medium pods of okra,
    chopped
6 to 8 pods of garlic, cut
½ bunch parsley, chopped
1 bunch green onions and
    tops, chopped

2 pounds cleaned deveined
    raw shrimp
1 pound fresh crab meat
½ cup shortening
1 bay leaf
½ cup flour
Salt
Pepper (red or black)
Filé

CONTINUED, CRAB & SHRIMP GUMBO

Cut chicken; salt and pepper and brown in small amount of shortening in large heavy Dutch oven. Remove brown chicken and make roux. This is done by melting shortening and adding ½ cup of flour and stirring constantly until dark brown, being careful not to burn. If there is the slightest indication of over browning, dispose of roux and start over. Add enough hot water to roux slowly, stirring rapidly, to prevent lumping, until thin and smooth. Fill Dutch oven half full of water and return chicken to cook until tender enough to remove all skin and bones; chop and return to Dutch oven. Now add celery, bell pepper, onions, bay leaf and garlic and cook these until vegetables are tender. Put shrimp, crab meat, parsley and green onions in last and cook about 15 minutes. Taste shrimp to be sure they are done. Season with salt, black pepper and red pepper to your own taste. Serve over bowls of rice with French bread or crackers. One-fourth teaspoon filé added to each bowl just before serving gives a good flavor.

Jim Graeber
Marks

TURKEY SOUP

SERVES: 12

Turkey carcass	Garlic and pepper to taste
½ cup chopped onion	1¼ cup uncooked rice
2 to 4 chicken bouillon cubes	1 tablespoon cornstarch
¾ cup parsley	½ cup cool water

Boil turkey carcass in large heavy Dutch oven, covered with water, with ½ cup chopped onion until meat is tender. Take the meat off bones and put aside. Add bouillon cubes, parsley, garlic salt and pepper to taste (other seasonings if you prefer). To broth add raw rice and cook until rice is done (usually floats to top) Mix cornstarch with water and add to broth and rice to thicken. Add chopped turkey and more seasoning if needed.

Stacy Falls
Sumner

Health Secret: Cheese is nutrient - dense; Cheddar, Swiss, Monterey Jack are high in protein and calcium, but also in fat and sodium.

CHEESE SANDWICH SURPRISES

My mother, Virginia Lowrance, adapted this recipe from Grandmother Bramlett's cheese sandwich by adding the chicken salad.

YIELD: 30 TO 35 SANDWICHES   OVEN 325°

1 pound sharp Cheddar
   cheese, grated
½ cup butter, softened
1 tablespoon Worcestershire
   sauce

1 teaspoon seasoned salt
1 tablespoon mayonnaise
1 teaspoon ground mustard
Your favorite chicken salad
1 loaf white sandwich bread

Blend first 6 ingredients in food processor. Prepare your favorite chicken salad. Cut crust from bread slices. Make chicken salad sandwiches; cut in half. Cover the entire sandwich with cheese mixture as if icing a cake. Arrange on greased cookie sheet and bake until slightly browned; about 10 minutes.

Jennie Neblett
Clarksdale

SLOPPY SUB

SERVES: 6

1 pound ground beef
1 pound hot sausage
1 pound jalapeño pasteur-
   ized processed cheese
   spread
1 tablespoon Worcestershire
   sauce

1 teaspoon oregano
Salt, pepper, garlic powder
   to taste
1 large loaf French bread

Brown meats; drain and add cheese. Cook until cheese melts. Add seasonings. Cut top from bread. Cut center out of bread (Toast and use as bread crumbs or croutons.) Fill bread with meat mixture. Put top back on bread. Wrap well in foil. Freeze or bake 30 minutes.

Family Secret: Add a small salad and you make a meal.

Gay Flowers
Mattson

Variation: Add 1 small chopped onion, 1 chopped bell pepper and 1 (4 ounce) can mushroom pieces to the meat while it browns.

Jane Webster
Clarksdale

PARTY CHICKEN SANDWICHES

SERVES: 8   OVEN: 350°

1 loaf thin sandwich bread	⅔ cup mayonnaise
2 cups chopped chicken	3 to 4 green onions, chopped
4 hard boiled eggs, chopped	Salt
½ small can chopped ripe	Pepper
olives	Dash of dry mustard

Using a 3 to 4 inch can or cookie cutter, cut rounds from bread. Each sandwich will need 3 slices. Combine remaining ingredients and spread between bread layers.

FROSTING:

2 (5 ounce) jars Old English	2 eggs, uncooked
Cheese, room temperature	½ cup margarine, softened

Beat until fluffy and consistency of frosting. Spread on top and sides of sandwich. Cover lightly and refrigerate for 24 hours. Place on jelly roll pan and cover with foil that has been sprayed with cooking spray. Bake 10-15 minutes. Topping will melt slightly and form a "puddle" around sandwiches.

Verne Kittell
Clarksdale

PO-BOY STEAK SANDWICH

SERVES: 4 TO ONE POUND OF MEAT

1 pound sirloin tip roast, sliced tissue paper thin at meat department	Provolone cheese or Swiss or mozzerella
Margarine	Submarine bun, French bread bun or steak bun
Chopped bell pepper, onions and/or fresh mushrooms	

Sauté slices of roast beef in skillet with pat of butter. Add bell pepper, onions and mushrooms (optional) to skillet and cook through. Remove sandwich filling. Spread margarine on buns. Heat steak bun, submarine bun, or French bread bun in skillet. Add cheese to hot bun. Remove from skillet, add meat portion to each bun. Garnish with mayonnaise, lettuce and tomato.

Family Secret: Serve with French fries or chips and kosher wedge pickle.

Mrs. Clifford P. Davis
Clarksdale

OPEN-FACE HAM SANDWICHES

YIELD: 8

1 (8 ounce) package cream
  cheese, softened
½ cup butter or margarine,
  softened
½ cup grated Parmesan
  cheese
1 teaspoon paprika
½ teaspoon dried whole
  oregano

½ teaspoon garlic powder
4 English muffins, split
8 slices cooked ham (about ¾
  pound)
8 slices tomato
8 slices onion
Fresh parsley sprigs

Combine cream cheese and butter; stir until smooth. Stir in cheese, paprika, oregano, and garlic powder. Spread two-thirds of mixture evenly over cut surface of English muffins; top each with a ham, onion, and tomato slice. Spoon remaining cheese mixture on center of tomato slice. Place on a baking sheet and broil until golden brown. Arrange sandwiches on platter and garnish with parsley.

Carolyn Webb
Sumner

MONTE CRISTO SANDWICHES

YIELD: 4

¼ cup mayonnaise
2¼ tablespoons prepared
  mustard
8 slices bread
4 (1 ounce) slices of cooked
  turkey
4 (1 ounce) slices of cooked
  ham
4 (1 ounce) slices Swiss
  cheese (low fat)

2 egg whites, at room
  temperature
3 eggs
½ cup sour cream
2 tablespoons milk
1 cup dry bread crumbs
Vegetable oil

Combine mayonnaise and mustard, spread on one side of each bread slice. Place one slice of each; turkey, ham, cheese, on top of 4 bread slices. Top the remaining bread slices. Cut each sandwich diagonally and secure with toothpicks. Beat egg whites until stiff. Set aside. Beat eggs, sour cream, and milk, fold in egg whites. Dip sandwich halves in batter. Coat with bread crumbs. Carefully lower coated sandwiches one at a time into deep hot oil (375°). Fry until golden brown; turn only once. Drain and remove toothpicks. Serve immediately.

Linda Hood
Duncan

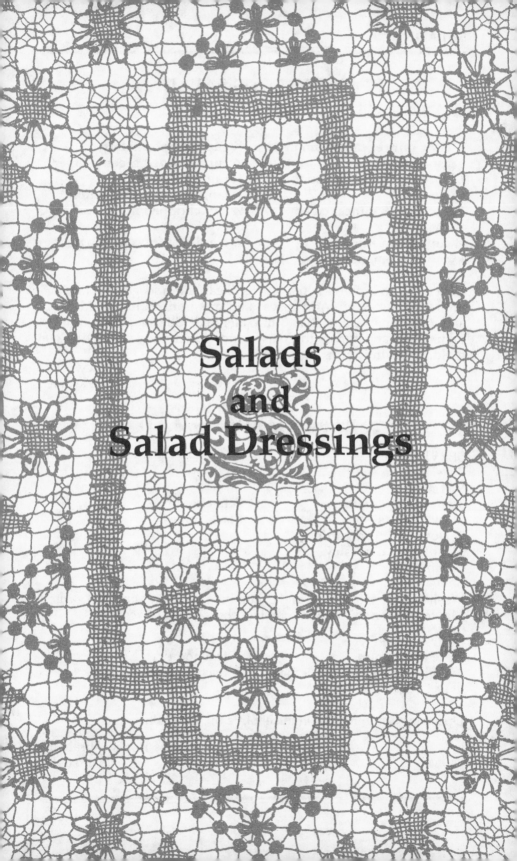

Salads
and
Salad Dressings

ASPARAGUS SALAD

SERVES: 12

1 (10¾ ounce) can cream of
  asparagus soup
1 package (3 ounce) lime
  gelatin
1 package (8 ounce) cream
  cheese
¼ cup lemon juice
1 cup mayonnaise

¾ cup chopped celery
½ cup chopped green pepper
1 can cut asparagus
1 tablespoon grated onion
½ cup chopped nuts
  (optional)
½ cup juice from asparagus

Heat soup to boiling. Remove from heat and add gelatin stirring until well dissolved. Add cheese and mix until melted. Add juice and mayonnaise and beat until blended. Stir in all remaining ingredients and turn into greased individual molds or one large mold. Chill until firm.

Lucy Frye
Clarksdale

ARABIC GARDEN SALAD

SERVES: 6

SALAD:
3 medium tomatoes
2 cucumbers
2 cloves minced garlic
1 tablespoon parsley,
  chopped

Feta cheese
Black olives

Wash and chop tomatoes and cucumbers. Add dressing and garlic. Mix together and top with parsley, cheese, and olives.

DRESSING:
Juice of 1 lemon
3 tablespoons olive oil - may
  use vegetable oil

1 teaspoon salt
1 teaspoon pepper

Dressing: Combine lemon juice, olive oil, and salt.

Yvonne Rossie Abraham
Clarksdale

SARA JANE'S ASPIC

SERVES: 6-8

1½ tablespoons gelatin
½ cup cold water
1 (10¾ ounce) can tomato
  soup
1 (8 ounce) package cream
  cheese, softened
½ to 1 cup mayonnaise
1 cup chopped celery

½ cup chopped green pepper
½ cup sliced green olives
1 tablespoon grated onion
2 tablespoons lemon juice
1 tablespoon Worcestershire
Dash hot sauce
Salt to taste

Soften gelatin in cold water. Heat soup to boiling point; add gelatin and dissolve completely. Slowly add to cream cheese. Stir until smooth. Cool; add mayonnaise gradually, then add all other ingredients. Pour in 9 x 13 inch (2 quart oblong) pyrex dish and chill until firm.

Family Secret: For variation add 1 pound cooked shrimp.

Louella G. Graves
Marks

BROCCOLI SALAD

SERVES: 10-12

1 bunch broccoli
½ to ⅔ cup sliced stuffed
  olives
1 small onion, chopped

¼ cup pickle relish
4 hard boiled eggs, chopped
1 teaspoon lemon juice
½ to ⅔ cup mayonnaise

Wash broccoli and cut into bite size pieces. Drain thoroughly on paper towels. Place in large bowl. Add other ingredients and mix lightly. Chill at least 12 hours. Keeps 3 or 4 days.

Family Secret: Makes a lot! Good! Can be served on lettuce or as a vegetable.

Lucy Frye
Clarksdale

Health Secret: One teaspoon of sugar has 16 calories; one teaspoon of fat, 40 calories.

MOLDED GAZPACHO

SERVES: 30 TO 40

10 envelopes unflavored
gelatin
2 (46 ounce) cans of
vegetable juice
3 or 4 tomatoes, peeled and
seeded
1 white onion, quartered
2 or 3 large cucumbers,
peeled and seeded
2¼ teaspoons of salt
½ bunch green onions,
chopped fine

1 teaspoon white pepper
1 teaspoon hot sauce
1 teaspoon Worcestershire
sauce
¼ cup lemon juice
¾ cup olive oil
¼ cup wine vinegar
2 teaspoon celery salt
Sour cream

In a large pan soften gelatin in 1 can of vegetable juice. Simmer until completely dissolved. In a blender purée tomatoes, white onion and cucumbers. Add to hot mixture with rest of ingredients. This recipe fills a 3 quart mold or a bundt pan. Chill until firm. Top each slice of salad with sour cream.

Family Secret: This recipe is so easy and quick and versatile, and I always have requests to make it. I have used it as an appetizer with crackers also. I usually make the whole recipe and take small servings to friends.

Carolyn Webb
Sumner

CUCUMBER SALAD

SERVES: 12 TO 15

7 cups cucumber, sliced thin
in food processor
1 large bell pepper, sliced
thin
1 large onion, sliced thin

3 tablespoons salt
1 cup white vinegar
2 cups sugar
1 tablespoon celery seed
3 teaspoons mustard seed

Sprinkle salt over sliced vegetables and let stand for 2 hours. Rinse 3 times in cold water and drain well. Bring vinegar, sugar, and seeds to boil together. Pour over vegetables and refrigerate. This will keep several weeks in the refrigerator. Use as a relish, on salad, or as a pickle.

Linda Dulaney
Clarksdale

GREEN BEAN SALAD

SERVES: 12

3 to 4 cans green beans
    (1 pound size)
5 to 6 ounces ranch style
    dressing

¼ cup toasted sunflower
    seeds

Drain beans thoroughly, place in bowl and toss with ranch dressing. Refrigerate overnight. When ready to serve, sprinkle with sunflower seeds. Quick and easy.

Family Secret: Good anytime, especially with a picnic or cool supper with baked ham and potato salad.

Nelle Gragg
Memphis, Tennessee

Add 2 (16 ounce) cans artichoke hearts, and 1 thinly sliced onion.

Mrs. Billy Frazer
Clarksdale

THREE BEAN SALAD

SERVES: 8-10

1 (16 ounce) can English peas
1 (16 ounce) can bean sprouts
1 (16 ounce) can French style
    green beans
1 cup chopped onion
1 cup chopped celery
1 cup diced pimento
1 cup sugar

1 cup white vinegar
1 cup vegetable oil
½ cup water
1 teaspoon salt
1 teaspoon basil
1 teaspoon oregano
1 teaspoon garlic salt

Drain the three cans of vegetables and leave in cans. Mix the onion, celery, and pimento together. Layer in a bowl green beans, then onion mixture, bean sprouts, onion mixture, English peas, and then onion mixture. Mix together in a boiler sugar, vinegar, oil, water, and salt. Heat and when the ingredients begin to boil add basil, oregano, and garlic salt. Boil food one minute. Pour over vegtable mixture. Chill, preferably overnight. Drain before serving.

Gayla Marley
Clarksdale

CONGEALED COLESLAW

SERVES: 6 TO 8

1 cup hot water
1 (3 ounce) package lemon or
   lime gelatin
½ cup cold water
2 teaspoons vinegar
½ cup mayonnaise
¼ teaspoon salt

Dash of black pepper
2 cups finely grated cabbage
2 teaspoons green pepper
   (chopped)
1 teaspoons onion (chopped)
½ teaspoon celery seed
½ cup grated carrot

Dissolve gelatin in hot water. Add next five ingredients, stir until well blended. Chill until soft set. Beat until fluffy and fold in cabbage, pepper, onion, celery seed and carrot. Pour into one quart mold and chill.

Peggy Beckham
Clarksdale

SPINACH SALAD AND
SALAD DRESSING

SERVES: 6-8

Fresh spinach (1 bag
   washed)-very dry
½ hard cooked egg per person

1 to 2 pieces bacon per
   person

Cook bacon until crisp: crumble. Slice eggs. Combine spinach, bacon and eggs. Toss with dressing.

DRESSING:
¾ cup oil (½ cup extra-virgin
   olive oil and ¼ cup
   vegetable oil)
¼ cup white vinegar
Juice of a whole large lemon

1 large clove garlic, mashed
   well or chopped finely
1 teaspoon salt
Coarse ground pepper to taste

Combine and shake.

Mrs. Harry Frazer (Penny)
Clarksdale

CRUNCHY GREEN PEA SALAD

SERVES: 4

1 (10 ounce) package frozen
  green peas
1 cup chopped fresh
  cauliflower
¼ cup diced green onion
2 tablespoons diced pimento
1 cup roasted cashews,
  macadamia nuts or
  sunflower seeds

¼ cup bacon bits
½ cup sour cream
1 cup prepared ranch-style
  dressing
½ teaspoon mustard,
  prepared
1 teaspoon garlic powder

Rinse peas in hot water; drain well. Combine vegetables, nuts and bacon with sour cream. Mix prepared dressing, mustard and garlic together. Pour over salad. Toss gently. Chill.

Nancy M. Daughdrill
Clarksdale

DINAH SHORE SALAD

My friend Judy Patterson exchanged recipes with Dinah Shore at dinner in Art Linkletter's home.

SERVES: 6

2 tablespoons red wine
  vinegar
5 tablespoons corn oil
1 tablespoon gourmet
  mustard
1 clove of garlic, minced
2 tablespoons scallions,
  chopped fine

2 teaspoons salt
Pinch of pepper
1 (12 ounce) box of
  mushrooms
1 bunch spinach
1 bunch Romaine salad
  greens

Mix dressing in the bottom of large salad bowl. Add mushrooms. Tear salad greens on top. Cover with plastic. Allow to stand overnight in refrigerator. Toss and serve.

Maggie Sherard
Sherard

SAINTS' CHICKEN SALAD

SERVES: 6 TO 8

4 cups cubed chicken
(4 whole breasts)
1 tablespoon grated onion
1 cup chopped celery
¼ cup sour cream
⅔ cup mayonnaise
1½ teaspoons salt

¼ teaspoon pepper
1 tablespoon tarragon
vinegar
4 hard boiled eggs (chopped)
½ cup chopped sweet pickles
or sweet pickle relish

Combine chicken, onion, celery. Mix sour cream, mayonnaise, salt, pepper, vinegar and chopped pickles. Combine both mixtures. Just before you serve, fold in hard boiled eggs.

St. George's Episcopal Day School
Clarksdale

ITALIAN PICNIC SALAD

SERVES: 10

SALAD:
1 (15 ounce) can artichokes
(cut each in several
sections)
4 ounces sliced salami (cut in
thin strips)
4 ounces ham (cut in thin
strips)
⅓ cup Parmesan cheese
1 cup coarsely grated
Cheddar cheese

1 cup coarsely grated
Montery Jack cheese
1 large bell pepper, chopped
¼ cup coarsely grated onion
Salt, pepper and hot sauce
to taste
8 ounces thin spaghetti
(cooked and drained)

DRESSING:
1 cup oil
⅓ cup vinegar
½ teaspoon oregano
½ teaspoon basil

1 clove garlic, crushed
½ teaspoon sugar
½ teaspoon salt
¼ teaspoon pepper

CONTINUED, ITALIAN PICNIC SALAD

PREPARATION INSTRUCTIONS:
Mix all salad ingredients together except hot sauce, salt, pepper, and spaghetti. Mix dressing ingredients together—you can do this several days ahead and refrigerate. Toss salad, spaghetti and dressing together. Can be prepared the day before using.

Family Secret: This salad can be used in place of potato salad at any time. It would also be good for lunch or supper along with a fresh fruit salad or tomato aspic. It is very good to take for a tail gate picnic at a ballgame.

Harvey Fiser
Clarksdale

TABBOULEH

SERVES: 4

½ cup fine cracked wheat
2 large tomatoes, diced
1 bunch green onions, chopped
4 bunches parsley, chopped
½ bunch mint, chopped or 2 tablespoons dried mint (optional)

½ cup olive oil
Juice of 3 lemons
1 teaspoon salt
½ teaspoon pepper

Wash cracked wheat. Drain and place in a large bowl. Add all chopped vegetables and mix well. Add oil, lemon juice, salt, and pepper. Allow cracked wheat to soak and absorb the juice (about 1 hour). Serve over fresh green lettuce. Eat with lettuce leaves, tender grape leaves, or with a fork. Makes a refreshing appetizer or picnic salad.

Elaine Daho
Clarksdale

ITALIAN TOMATO SALAD

SERVES: 6

6 firm tomatoes
1 teaspoon dried basil
¼ teaspoon marjoram and garlic powder

Salt and pepper to taste
¼ cup olive oil

Cut tomatoes into wedges, add seasonings and oil. Toss gently and refrigerate for 1 hour.

Theresa Malatesta
Shaw

CRAB MEAT SALAD

SERVES: 6

2 (6½ ounce) cans crab meat
2 cups cooked rice, cooled
1 (8 ounce) can green peas,
   drained
1½ cups finely diced celery

¼ cup sliced pimento
1 cup mayonnaise
1½ tablespoons lemon juice
1 teaspoon salt
½ teaspoon pepper

Mix crabmeat, rice, peas, celery, and pimentos. Blend remaining ingredients. Pour over crab meat mixture and toss lightly. Adjust seasonings, if necessary. Chill and serve.

Family Secret: You may substitute 12 ounces of fresh or frozen cooked shrimp for the crab meat.

Patricia Simpson
Clarksdale

GERMAN POTATO SALAD

SERVES: 5 TO 6

½ pound bacon (10 to 12
   slices)
½ cup chopped onion
2 to 3 tablespoons all
   purpose flour
¾ cup sugar

1½ teaspoons salt
1 teaspoon celery seed
Dash of pepper
½ cup vinegar (white)
1 cup water
6 cups sliced cooked potatoes

In an iron skillet, cook bacon till crisp; drain and crumble, reserving ¼ cup fat. Cook onion in reserved fat till tender. Blend in flour, sugar, salt, celery seed, and a dash of pepper; add vinegar and 1 cup water; cook and stir until thick and bubbly. Add bacon and potatoes. Heat thoroughly tossing lightly. Serve immediately or keep it warm in the skillet and serve it later. It must be served warm.

Family Secret: This is a great side dish with a good sandwich.

Mrs. Jane Rutz
Lyon

SUMMER SALAD

SERVES: 6 TO 8

3 medium fresh tomatoes
Lettuce cups
1 (16 ounce) can whole green
  beans

Italian dressing
Homemade mayonnaise

Arrange sliced tomatoes or wedges of tomatoes on lettuce. Sprinkle with salt and pepper. Place green beans that have been marinated overnight in Italian dressing on tomatoes, and top with a dollop of homemade mayonnaise

So easy and delicious! Can be made ahead.

Family Secret: Perfect way to show off your home grown 'maters.

Gay Flowers
Clarksdale

CONGEALED APPLESAUCE SALAD

SERVES: 8-10

1 (3 ounce) package cherry
  gelatin
1 (3 ounce) package
  strawberry gelatin
2 cups boiling water

1 (8 ounce) cream cheese,
  softened
2 (1 pound) cans applesauce
1 (10 ounce) cola drink

Dissolve gelatin in boiling water. Add cream cheese, stirring to dissolve. Add remaining ingredients and refrigerate to congeal.

Margaret Sandifer
Clarksdale

FROZEN CRANBERRY SALAD

SERVES: 10 TO 12

6 ounces cream cheese,
  softened
2 teaspoons mayonnaise

2 (16 ounce) cans whole
  cranberries
½ cup chopped pecans

Mix all ingredients. Pour in 3 quart oblong dish. Freeze. Remove from freezer 5 minutes before cutting.

Mary Poole
Clarksdale

PINEAPPLE CONGEALED SALAD

SERVES: 15 TO 20

1 (20 ounce) can crushed
  pineapple, drained and
  juice reserved
1 (6 ounce) package lemon
  gelatin
1 (8 ounce) package of cream
  cheese, softened
2 (2 ounce) jars of chopped
  pimento

1 cup finely chopped celery
1 cup chopped pecans
1 cup mayonnaise
1 pinch of salt
1 pint whipping cream,
  whipped

Drain pineapple. Add enough water to juice to make three cups. Heat juice mixture to boiling and add gelatin to dissolve. Soften cream cheese by adding a small amount of the juice mixture and beat. Add the remainder of the juice mixture and mix well. Refrigerate until partially congealed then add the remaining ingredients by stirring gently. Fold in whipped cream. Pour into a three quart pyrex dish to continue the congealing process. Cut in squares to serve.

Family Secret: For a salad lover, this is really satisfying as a complete meal along with cheese toast or your favorite cracker.

Donna Dees
Clarksdale

ORANGE RICE SALAD

SERVES: 10 TO 12

¼ pound snow peas
3 cups cooked brown rice
2 to 3 green onions, sliced
1 cup celery, chopped
⅛ cup fresh parsley, chopped
1 cup green pepper, chopped
1 (8 ounce can) water
   chestnuts, sliced
1 cup diced pineapple, fresh
   or canned and drained

1 unpeeled apple, seeded,
   and chopped
1½ cups red or green grapes,
   halved
¾ cup raisins
½ cup nuts (cashews, peanuts,
   or pecans)
¼ cup sesame seeds, toasted

Steam snow peas for 2 to 3 minutes. Rinse under cold water. Drain. Combine the other ingredients in a large bowl. Add nuts and seeds just before serving.

DRESSING:
¼ cup orange juice
   concentrate, thawed
¼ cup lite mayonnaise
1 teaspoon fresh ginger,
   chopped

1 to 2 teaspoons curry
1 teaspoon grated orange
   peel
1 clove garlic, minced

To prepare dressing: Blend together orange juice concentrate, mayonnaise and spices. Pour over salad and toss gently, blending well.

Emily Cooper
Clarksdale

MONTICELLO DRESSING

YIELD: 1½ CUPS

1 small clove of garlic
   (crushed)
1 teaspoon salt
½ teaspoon white pepper

⅓ cup olive oil
⅓ cup sesame oil
⅓ cup tarragon or wine
   vinegar

Combine the above ingredients and place in a covered jar or bottle. Shake well. Chill.

Mrs. Inger H. Flautt
Sumner

ITALIAN SALAD DRESSING

¼ teaspoon paprika
¼ teaspoon dry mustard
½ teaspoon salt
½ teaspoon fresh ground
    black pepper
1 clove garlic (peeled and
    rubbed on wooden salad
    bowl before salad greens
    are added)

¼ cup red wine vinegar
¾ cup olive oil (or good corn
    oil)

Mix above ingredients and refrigerate. Can be stored in refrigerator. Always use a variety of raw vegetables in salad such as yellow squash, red onions, mushrooms, artichoke hearts, and tomato. Mix raw veggies with dressing in bottom of bowl and let marinate for one hour or longer. Mix two or more types of lettuce for a pretty salad. Raw spinach is great for color and flavor. A sprinkle of freshly grated Parmesan or Romano cheese is a nice touch. Do not toss until ready to serve.

Toni Malvessi Hardin
Duncan

NANNIE BRAMLETT'S
1000 ISLAND DRESSING

I never think of Sunday lunch as a child that I don't remember Nannie's head of lettuce salad topped with this marvelous salad dressing.

YIELD: 2 CUPS

1 cup mayonnaise
2 tablespoons chili sauce
2 tablespoons catsup
2 teaspoons mustard

2 hard boiled eggs, chopped
2 tablespoons chopped bell
    pepper
3 tablespoons chopped celery

Mix all ingredients together and chill. Will keep grand in refrigerator.

Gay Flowers
Dublin

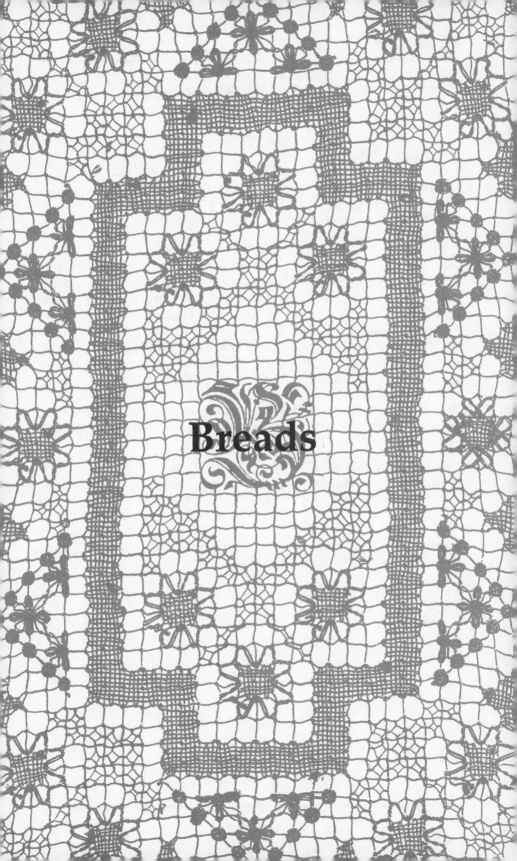

Breads

CREAM CHEESE BRAIDS

YIELD: 4 BRAIDS   OVEN: 375°

DOUGH:

1 cup sour cream	2 packages dry yeast
½ cup sugar	½ cup warm water
1 teaspoon salt	2 eggs, beaten
½ cup butter or margarine, melted	4 cups all purpose flour

Heat sour cream over low heat; stir in sugar, salt and butter and cool to lukewarm. Sprinkle yeast over warm water in large mixing bowl, stirring until yeast dissolves. Add sour cream mixture, eggs and flour; mix well. Cover tightly and refrigerate overnight. The next day divide dough into 4 equal parts, roll out each part on well floured surface into 12 inch by 8 inch rectangle. Spread ¼ cream cheese mixture on each rectangle. Roll up jelly-roll style, beginning at long sides. Pinch edges together and place on greased cookie sheet seam side down. Slit each roll at 2 inch intervals ⅔ way through the dough to resemble a braid. Cover and let rise in warm place until double in size (about 1 hour). Bake 12 to 15 minutes until golden brown. Spread with glaze mixture while warm.

CREAM CHEESE FILLING:

2 (8 ounce) packages cream cheese, softened	1 egg, beaten
¾ cup sugar	⅛ teaspoon salt
	2 teaspoons vanilla

Combine cream cheese and sugar in small mixing bowl. Add egg, salt and vanilla. Mix well.

GLAZE:

2 cups powdered sugar	2 teaspoons vanilla
¼ cup milk	

Combine, stirring to dissolve lumps.

Louella G. Graves
Marks

HOT ROLLS

YIELD: 7 DOZEN   OVEN: 350°

4 cups sweet milk   8 cups flour, divided
1 cup shortening   1 tablespoon salt
1 cup sugar   1½ teaspoons soda
1 package yeast   2 teaspoons baking powder

Heat milk, shortening and sugar to boiling point. (I use microwave).
Set aside until lukewarm. Then add yeast. Beat in 4 cups of flour
and let stand 2 hours at room temperature. Add salt, soda, baking
powder and other 4 cups of flour. Store in refrigerator until you are
ready to bake rolls. About 2½ hours before baking, roll out rolls and
dip in butter, fold and place on baking tray. Cover them while they
rise. Bake about 15 minutes.

Family Secret: Very yeasty!

Patsy Maclin
Clarksdale

ITALIAN DRESSING BREAD

SERVES: 6 TO 8   OVEN: 350°

1 loaf frozen bread   1 package dry Italian salad
½ cup margarine, melted   dressing mix

Thaw bread. Mix dressing and margarine together. Pinch bread
into balls. Roll balls in butter mixture and drop into bundt pan.
Pour remaining mixture over balls. Let rise until bread is at top of
pan, about 3 hours. Cook until brown 30 to 35 minutes.

Barbara Agostinelli
Lyon

SWEDISH NUT ROLLS

This was a traditional Christmas treat that we enjoyed for breakfast, for dessert or snacks, and to give as gifts. While I was in college, Mama would always send some right after Thanksgiving. They were a hit in the dorm and kept us going as we studied for exams.

YIELD: 125-150 SMALL

OVEN: 350°

FILLING:
3 cups sugar
3 to 4 tablespoons melted margarine or butter
3 cups finely ground nuts

⅓ cup cream
Grated rind of 3 lemons
3 teaspoons vanilla

Mix all ingredients together and refrigerate overnight.

DOUGH:
4½ cups flour
½ cup sugar
¾ teaspoon salt
½ pound margarine or butter (2 sticks)

Grated rind of 1 lemon
2 packages yeast, dissolved in ¼ cup lukewarm milk
½ cup sour cream
3 eggs (reserve 1 egg white)

Note: May need another egg white to brush on nut rolls. Sift the flour, salt and sugar into a large mixing bowl. Cut in butter or margarine as for pie crust. When it is finely crumbled, add lemon rind, dissolved yeast, sour cream, and the beaten eggs (minus one egg white). Knead until the dough comes away from the bowl without sticking. Cover, and place in the refrigerator overnight. The next morning, divide the dough into equal portions: cut basic dough in half, then quarters, then quarters into 4 wedges each. Return to refrigerator, removing only one wedge at a time. Roll each to form a 6 inch round and spread with filling. Cut the round into 8 to 10 wedge - shaped pieces like a pie. Roll up each wedge from the outer rim of the circle to the center. Brush the top with beaten egg white and sprinkle with sugar. Place on a greased baking sheet and allow to double in size at room temperature (about 1 hour). Bake until golden brown.

Marilyn Young
Clarksdale

BUTTER COFFEE CAKES

YIELD: 3 CAKES   OVEN: 350°

1 cup brown sugar
1 cup chopped pecans
2 teaspoons cinnamon
1 box yellow butter cake mix
½ cup margarine, softened

1 (8 ounce) carton sour cream
4 eggs
1 (6 ounce) package vanilla
   instant pudding mix
¼ cup oil

Grease and flour 3 (8 inch) round pans. Combine sugar, pecans and cinnamon. Sprinkle each pan lightly with ½ of mixture. Combine remaining ingredients. Pour evenly into pans. Sprinkle rest of dry mixture on top and bake 30 to 40 minutes. May freeze in pans.

Georgia Wilson
Clarksdale

BRAN MUFFINS

YIELD: 18 MUFFINS   OVEN: 425°

2¼ cups bran cereal
2½ cups all-purpose flour
1½ cups sugar
1 teaspoon salt

2½ teaspoons baking soda
½ cup oil
2 cups nonfat buttermilk
3 egg whites

Mix ingredients together with a spoon. Fill regular size muffin tin (which has been sprayed with a non-stick cooking spray) ¾ full. Bake for 17 minutes. Serve warm. This mixture may be kept in an air tight container in the refrigerator for several weeks.

Family Secret: Our family loves these. I adapted it from an old recipe to make them lower in fat and cholesterol.

Mrs. Rick Parsons
Vance

BANANA MUFFINS

YIELD: 12 LARGE OR 24 SMALL   OVEN: 350°

½ cup butter, softened
1 cup sugar
1 egg, beaten
1 cup mashed banana
1½ cups less 2 tablespoons
  all-purpose flour

1 teaspoon soda in 1
  tablespoon boiling water
1 teaspoon nutmeg
1 teaspoon vanilla

Cream butter and sugar and add beaten egg. Add rest of ingredients.
Bake about 20 minutes.

Mrs. Walter W. Thompson
Clarksdale

JACK-O-LANTERN PUMPKIN BREAD

*We always wait until Halloween Day to carve our jack-o-
lantern. Then, after he has served his purpose on the porch, he
is washed thoroughly and placed in a slow oven (300°) until he
collapses. The next morning I scoop out the soft pulp (the string
part and seeds were removed at carving time). A few seconds in
the food processor and old Jack now is pumpkin that can be used
in bread, pies, cake, etc.*

YIELD: 4 (1 POUND) CANS   OVEN: 350°

3 cups sugar
1 cup oil
4 eggs
2 cups mashed pumpkin (or
  No. 2 can)
¾ cup orange juice
3½ cups flour

1½ teaspoons salt
2 teaspoons soda
1 teaspoon nutmeg
1 teaspoon cinnamon
1 cup raisins
1 cup pecans

Cream oil and sugar. Add eggs one at a time, beating after each
addition. Add pumpkin and mix. Sift dry ingredients and add them
alternately with orange juice. Add raisins and pecans. Grease and
flour 4 (1 pound) coffee cans or 4 small loaf pans. Fill half full with
mixture. Bake for 1 hour. Remove from oven and let cool for 10
minutes. Remove from can and wrap in plastic wrap.

Sherry Donald
Clarksdale

JOYCE'S MEXICAN CORNBREAD

SERVES: 8 TO 10   OVEN: 450°

MEAT MIXTURE:

1½ pounds ground round or
  ground sirloin
½ pound hot sausage
½ cup chopped onions
½ cup chopped bell peppers
½ teaspoon garlic powder

1 teaspoon chili powder
½ teaspoon seasoned salt
1 tablespoon
  Worcestershire sauce
1 tablespoon soy sauce

Sauté meat and other ingredients until meat is browned and onions are clear.

CORNBREAD MIXTURE:

2 packages Mexican
  cornbread mix
4 eggs
1 (8 ounce) carton French
  onion dip

1½ cups frozen whole kernel
  corn
1 to 1½ cups buttermilk

Mix together as for cornbread. Fold meat mixture into cornbread mixture.** Grease 9 x 13 inch pan. Pour mixture into pan and bake until browned (30 to 35 minutes). Cut into squares and enjoy! **You can sprinkle 1 cup shredded Cheddar cheese over mixture just before pouring into pan to bake.

Joyce W. Edmondsom
Clarksdale

GRANDMOTHER'S CORNBREAD

SERVES: 9   OVEN: 425°

1 cup yellow meal
1 cup sifted flour
2 tablespoons sugar
½ teaspoon salt

4 teaspoons baking powder
2 eggs, lightly beaten
1 cup milk
¼ cup oil

Spray a 9 x 9 inch heavy skillet with non-stick spray and put in preheated oven. Sift dry ingredients into medium size bowl. Add eggs, milk and oil. Beat until smooth. Remove skillet from oven and pour batter into it. Bake 20 to 25 minutes.

Emily Cooper
Clarksdale

HEATON'S PECAN BROWN BREAD

YIELD: 1 LARGE LOAF   OVEN: 350°

¼ cup sugar
3 cups whole wheat flour
1 teaspoon salt
3 teaspoons baking soda

1 to 1½ cups chopped pecans
2 cups buttermilk
½ cup molasses
1 tablespoon butter, melted

Mix all dry ingredients. Mix milk, molasses and butter; add to first mixture. Pour into large greased loaf pan. Bake 45 minutes.

Chris Heaton
Clarksdale

WHOLE WHEAT ROLLS

YIELD: 6 DOZEN   OVEN 375° TO 400°

1 quart milk (may use low
fat)
1 cup lard (do not substitute
shortening or oil)
1 cup sugar
1 package yeast

¼ cup warm (not hot) water
7 cups pre-sifted plain flour
2 cups whole wheat flour
1 tablespoon salt
½ teaspoon baking soda

Scald 1 quart milk, lard and sugar in double boiler. (I use microwave on medium for 18 to 20 minutes.) Pour into a big bowl and cool. Add yeast to water and dissolve. Add yeast to milk mixture along with 7 cups of flour. Cover with foil and let rise several hours or until doubled. Punch down and add 2 cups whole wheat flour, salt and baking soda. Mix well, cover and refrigerate overnight. To roll out rolls, knead several times. Sprinkle surface with flour. Cut out rolls and brush with melted margarine. Fold in half. This mixture keeps several days in the refrigerator. May use as needed.

Toni M. Hardin
Duncan

HUSH PUPPIES

YIELD: 2 DOZEN

1 cup onion, chopped fine
1 cup sharp cheese, grated
1 cup plain corn meal
1½ teaspoons salt

1 teaspoon black pepper
1 teaspoon red pepper
1 cup boiling water

Mix all above ingredients in a bowl, except water, until well blended. Pour boiling water over and stir until moist. Dividing with a tablespoon, pat dough flat and make a hole in the center (like a doughnut). Drop in hot grease and cook until brown. Drain on paper. Serve warm.

Jewell Graeber
Marks

ICE BOX BISCUITS

YIELD: 1 TO 2 DOZEN   OVEN: 350°

2 cups flour
4 teaspoons baking powder
1 teaspoon salt

5 tablespoons shortening
1 cup sweet milk

Cut shortening into dry ingredients. Add milk and knead a few times. Roll out on floured board and cut with biscuit cutter. Place biscuits on ungreased cookie sheet and freeze for 30 minutes or until hard. Remove and package in freezer bags and return to freezer. When ready to use, remove from freezer and let thaw 30 minutes. Bake 20 minutes.

Family Secret: These are real short and crispy! Will keep indefinitely in freezer.

Mrs. Graham Bramlett
Clarksdale

PEPPERONI BREAD

SERVES: 8 TO 10   OVEN: 350°

1 loaf frozen bread dough
4 ounces pizza sauce or
  spaghetti sauce
4 ounces mozzarella cheese,
  grated

4 ounces Cheddar cheese,
  grated
4 ounces pepperoni, sliced

Thaw out bread dough. Roll out to approximately 10 by 14 inch rectangle. Down the center place ½ pizza sauce, ½ pepperoni, ½ of both cheeses. Fold one of the ends over the center portion. Repeat the filling. Fold the remaining dough over the filling and seal ends and side with fingers. Bake until golden brown. Brush with melted margarine to soften shell.

Kathy Davis
Clarksdale

WOODY'S ROLLS

YIELD: APPROXIMATELY 5 DOZEN   OVEN: 400°

1 cup shortening
2 eggs, beaten
½ cup sugar
1 cup milk, scalded

1 package yeast
1 cup lukewarm water
2 teaspoons salt
6 cups flour (plain)

Mix the eggs, shortening and sugar together. Mix in warm milk. Combine yeast and lukewarm water. Add flour with salt to egg mixture. Add yeast and stir until well mixed. Cover and put in refrigerator. (Let it stay overnight). Take out as much as you please. Form rolls and let rise for 1 to 1½ hours. Bake 10-12 minutes.

Family Secret: Rain or shine, they will rise.

Mrs. Willie M. Herron
Clarksdale

SMITH LAKE BREAD

SERVES: 8   OVEN: 350°

1 loaf French bread   Poppy seed
1 stick butter, melted   1 package sliced Swiss
½ cup onions   cheese
1½ tablespoons mustard   Bacon slices
Dash red pepper sauce

Slice the top off bread and shave sides. Slice the remaining loaf into slices, but not all the way through. Melt butter and add onions, mustard, and dash of red pepper sauce. Brush butter on each slice and sprinkle with poppy seeds between slices. Lay cheese and bacon on top. Bake until bacon is done, or about 20 minutes.

Linda Dulaney
Clarksdale

SPOON ROLLS

YIELD: 2 DOZEN   OVEN: 350°

1 package dry yeast   1 egg
2 cups very warm water   4 cups unsifted self rising
1½ sticks margarine, melted   flour
¼ cup sugar

Place yeast in 2 cups water. Cream margarine and sugar together in large bowl. Add egg and cream a little more. Add yeast and water mixture, stir and add flour. Mix well with electric mixer. Place in air tight bowl. Keep refrigerated. To cook, drop by spoonful into well greased muffin tins. Bake about 20 minutes. Will keep in refrigerator about 1 week.

Mrs. Jeff Clark
Tutwiler

JENNY'S HERB ROLLS

YIELD: 24-36   OVEN: 425°

½ cup butter (I use a little
  less), melted
1½ teaspoons parsley flakes
½ teaspoon dill weed
1 tablespoon onion flakes

2 tablespoons Parmesan
  cheese
1 (10 or 11 ounce) can
  refrigerator buttermilk
  biscuits

Add seasonings to melted butter. Cut biscuits into halves or fourths
and swish around in the herb butter to coat on all sides. Bake for 12
to 15 minutes.

Baby Doll Peacock Walker (Mrs. Ben. Jr.)
Tribbett

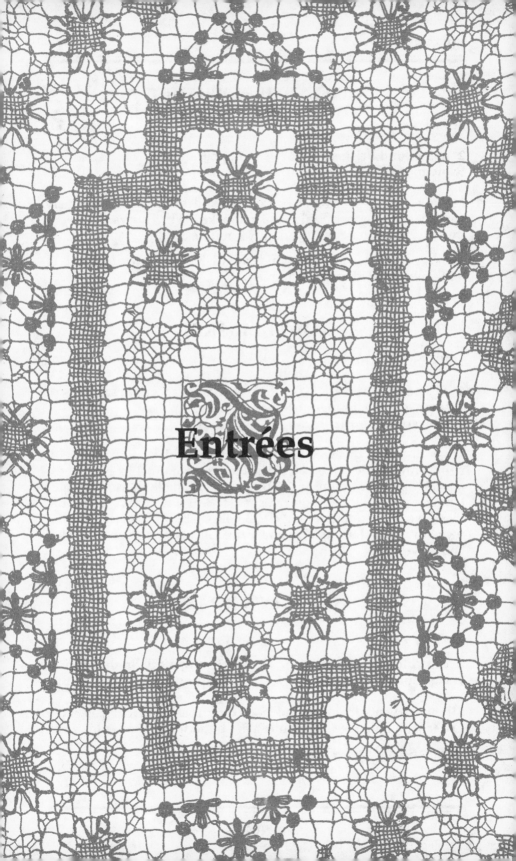

Entrées

ITALIAN BEEF BRISKET

SERVES: 6   OVEN: 350°

2 to 3 pound brisket   **Pepper**
Ripieno stuffing (Page 173)

Make a pocket in side of brisket and fill with "P". Generously sprinkle with pepper. Seal in foil and bake 2½ to 3 hours. Slice very thin (½ inch) after cooling about 30 minutes.

Family Secret: It is really a wonderful dish to serve with a good oil and vinegar salad and fresh bread.

Celeste Wise
Clarksdale

ROAST BRISKET

SERVES: 8 TO 10   OVEN: 350°

4 to 5 pound brisket   **Salt, pepper, garlic salt to**
1 large onion, chopped   **taste**
1 tablespoon shortening

Wash and dry the well trimmed brisket and season with salt, pepper and garlic salt on all sides. Place in pan (9 x 13 x 2½ inches) fat side up. Sauté onions in 1 tablespoon vegetable shortening until tender - not brown. Spoon over roast. Seal with heavy duty foil. Place in oven and forget for 2½ to 3 hours. The brisket will make its own gravy which is delicious over rice. Slice across grain of brisket and serve.

Flora Hirsberg
Clarksdale

PARSON'S ROAST

OVEN: 325°

2 cups bloody mary mix   **1 envelope dry onion soup**
1 cup Burgundy wine   **2 heaping tablespoons flour**

Mix ingredients together and pour over roast (any cut you like). Cover with foil: bake 20 minutes per pound for medium rare roast.

Family Secret: I use a sirloin tip.

Carlisle Parsons
Vance

RARE ROAST BEEF

SERVES: 10 TO 12   OVEN: 500°

8 pound sirloin tip roast   Garlic powder
Salt   Worcestershire sauce
Pepper   Kitchen Bouquet

Allow roast to sit at room temperature for 45 minutes to 1 hour. Rub roast with spices. The amounts to your taste. Spray shallow roasting pan with no-stick cooking spray and place meat in it. Brown meat in hot oven for 15 minutes. Turn off oven and let cool; then bake 15 minutes to the pound at 250°. For 8 pounds, almost 2 hours. No water, no lid.

Laurenze Cooper Bouldin
(Mrs. Marshall Bouldin, Jr.)
Clarksdale

CHILI

SERVES: 10

3 pounds ground chuck   Salt and black pepper to taste
2 large onions, chopped   4 (10½ ounce) cans tomato
4 tablespoons cumin   soup
2 tablespoons paprika   4 soup cans of water
10 tablespoons chili powder   2 (16 ounce) cans red kidney
½ teaspoon red pepper   beans
   (cayenne)

Brown meat; add onions and next 5 ingredients. Cook until onions are limp. Add soup, water, and beans. Simmer 2 to 3 hours.

George Black
Clarksdale

Health Secret: Many recipes call for more fat than is necessary. Try using only one - half the amount recommended. You may need to add wine, fruit juice or broth to replace some of the moisture.

BAKED KIBBIE

SERVES: 6   OVEN: 350°

KIBBIE:

1 scant cup cracked wheat, #1 size

1 pound Kibbie Meat (This is top round steak with all fat trimmed, ground three times. Meat should be very red with little or no fat.)

1 small onion, grated (Use food processor if available. You do not want to have any chopped pieces, just juice.)

Salt and pepper to taste

½ cup melted margarine or butter

Measure wheat and put in medium size bowl. Run cold water over it several times, rinsing several times. You may lose a little wheat when rinsing. Leave enough water in bowl to more than cover wheat. Sit aside and put timer on 20 minutes for wheat to soak. While wheat is soaking, sauté onions in a little margarine in skillet. When soft, add meat for filling and brown, crumbling as you brown it. Add chopped nuts and stir well into mixture. Add salt, pepper, and a little mint (optional) to taste. By this time, wheat should be ready. Put kibbie meat in large bowl. Take a handful of wheat and squeeze water out using your hands. Knead this into meat a handful at a time, until all wheat has been added. Add grated onion and mix well with hands. Add salt and pepper to taste. Seasoning is very important. You will have to taste this. Next, put several ice cubes in small bowl and add water. Stir around until very cold. Add a little ice water to the kibbie and mix until moist. Butter your 8½ x 11 inch casserole dish. Taking half of the kibbie mixture, make 1 layer of raw kibbie. Take the crumbled filling and sprinkle on top of this layer. Take a handful of kibbie meat and pat it down, placing in sections on top of filling, until top layer is smooth and filling is covered. You can dip hands in the ice water for easy patting. Next, score the casserole in diamond shapes or squares or rectangles, being sure to cut through all layers. Melt margarine and drizzle in cracks and around sides. This will keep the dish moist. Bake for 30 minutes.

FILLING:

1 to 1½ pounds ground round or lean chuck

1 small onion, chopped

½ to ¾ cup chopped nuts: pecans, cashews, or pine nuts

Salt and pepper

Dried mint if available

CONTINUED, BAKED KIBBIE:

Family Secret: Serve Baked Kibbie with broccoli, green beans, or squash, salad with oil and vinegar and lemon juice dressing, pocket bread or French bread.

Georgia Abraham Wilson
Clarksdale

KIBBIE

SERVES: 4 TO 6

2 pounds lean beef
2 medium onions, chopped
3 cups fine cracked wheat

2 tablespoons salt
1 teaspoon pepper

Remove all fat from meat and cut in cubes. Grind the meat finely twice. Grind onions once. Mix with ground meat and grind one more time. Wash cracked wheat and drain water by cupping hands and squeezing out all moisture. Mix with ground meat and onions, salt, and pepper. Grind or knead the mixture twice, adding water little by little until you get the kibbie dough soft and smooth. Form kibbie dough into patties and fry for 5 to 10 minutes in hot deep oil, or until golden brown.

Family Secret: Serve with salad or Tabbouleh.

Elaine Daho
Clarksdale

MEAT LOAF

SERVES: 6   OVEN: 350°

2 pounds ground beef
2 eggs
⅓ cup catsup
½ cup water
1 envelope onion soup mix
⅓ cup cooked rice

½ cup diced celery
1 cup soft Italian style bread crumbs or more if needed to make loaf firmer
1 (8 ounce) jar mushroom spaghetti sauce

Mix first 8 ingredients and shape into individual loaves and cover with a jar of mushroom spaghetti sauce. Bake with a little water in pyrex dish until done. Can be frozen but leave off spaghetti sauce until ready to cook.

Kathaleen D. Dulaney
Clarksdale

JOHNNY BIGATTI

While enjoying a football week-end in New Orleans during my college years, a fraternity brother, Tad Trowbridge, invited a few of us to his home for dinner. His mother served Johnny Bigatti. I enjoyed it so much that I asked Mrs. Trowbridge for the recipe.

SERVES: 12 TO 15   OVEN: 350°

2 pounds lean ground beef
2 medium onions, chopped
1 green pepper, chopped
2 (10½ ounce) cans cream of tomato soup
1 (16 ounce) can niblet corn
1 (4 ounce) can sliced mushrooms
Salt and pepper to taste

1 teaspoon Worcestershire sauce
2 cups (1 pound) grated Cheddar cheese, divided
8 to 10 ounces medium noodles, cooked and drained
Slivered almonds

Brown and drain ground beef. Return to pan. Add onions and pepper. Cover and cook until vegetables are soft. Add next 5 ingredients plus 1 cup cheese; add noodles. Mix well. Spray a 3 quart casserole with non-stick cooking spray. Pour in beef-noodle mixture and top with remaining cheese and almonds. Bake about one hour or until it bubbles around the sides.

Family Secret: To lower the fat content reduce the meat and cheese by half and increase the noodles and vegetables.

Wert Cooper
Clarksdale

TAMALE PIE

SERVES: 6 TO 8   OVEN: 350°

1 pound ground beef
1 large green pepper, chopped
1 medium onion, chopped
1 tablespoon chili powder
¼ teaspoon cumin
Salt and pepper to taste

1 (20 ounce) can tomatoes and juice, broken up
1 (12 ounce) can niblet corn
1 (4 ounce) can ripe olives
½ cup yellow corn meal
½ cup cold water

Brown ground beef in large skillet and cook. Add next six ingredients. Stir in corn meal and cold water and cook until thickened. Put in greased 7½ x 11 inch casserole. Cover with topping.

CONTINUED, TAMALE PIE:

TOPPING:
¼ pound grated Cheddar   1 cup milk
  cheese   ½ cup corn meal

Mix all ingredients in saucepan. Heat over low heat until thick, stirring constantly. May be cooked in microwave.

Fran Mullens
Lyon

PASTITSO
(MACARONI & MEAT CASSEROLE)

This recipe was one of the treasures my mother brought with her when she came to America from Greece.

SERVES: 40   OVEN: 350°

MACARONI MIXTURE:
1 cup butter, melted and   1½ pounds elbow macaroni
  separated   Salt and pepper (to taste)
1½ pounds ground chuck

Melt ½ cup butter in skillet and add ground chuck. Stir until brown, adding salt and pepper to taste. Set this mixture aside. Boil macaroni until almost done, drain well, and put in large bowl. Stir in other ½ cup melted butter. Set aside. Grease bottom and sides of pan (11 x 14 x 2 inch). Put ½ macaroni mixture into pan. Then cover macaroni with all of ground chuck mixture and top with remaining macaroni. Set aside.

CREMA SAUCE:
1 cup butter, melted   9 eggs
3 cups milk   1 pound Parmesan cheese

Beat eggs until smooth, then stir in melted butter and milk. Slowly mix in Parmesan cheese. Mix all ingredients well and spread over macaroni mixture, making sure it goes through the mixture. Bake 1 hour or until brown. Let stand about 15 minutes; then cut in squares.

Family Secret: This may be frozen and warmed again to serve.

Jean Ellington
Memphis, Tennessee

WEEZIE'S SPAGHETTI

YIELD: 12 TO 14 PINTS

½ cup butter or margarine
4 inch square salt meat,
  chopped fine in processor
8 medium onions
1 whole stalk celery
8 carrots (1 pound)
Small bunch parsley, stems
  removed
3 pounds ground beef (or 2
  pounds ground beef and 1
  pound chicken gizzards
  and livers)

2 (16 ounce) cans tomatoes
6 (6 ounce) cans tomato paste
3 packages dried mushrooms
2 to 3 garlic buds
Salt and pepper
3 to 4 bay leaves
Pinch rosemary
6 to 8 cups water

Chop onions, celery, carrots and parsley in food processor. Brown ground beef in skillet. Transfer to big pot. Wash skillet, then melt margarine and sauté salt meat. Add onions and other vegetables and sauté. Add all ingredients to large pot except water. Boil dried mushrooms in water for several minutes. Add after draining. Cook slowly for about an hour, stirring frequently. Add water and cook for at least another hour. The longer, the better. Add more water, ½ cup at a time, as necessary. Serve with prepared pasta and top with grated Parmesan cheese.

Family Secret: May be served with Italian meatballs.

Toni Malvezzi Hardin
Duncan

BEEF STROGANOFF

SERVES: 6

2 pounds sirloin
2 sticks butter
½ pint whipping cream
1 (16 ounce) carton sour
  cream

3 (4 ounce) cans button
  mushrooms
1 teaspoon garlic salt
1 large package egg noodles

Brown cut up meat in butter. Add whipping cream, sour cream, salt, pepper and garlic salt. Let this simmer on top of stove for 2 hours. Just before serving, cook noodles. Pour stroganoff over noodles and serve.

Sherry M. Eason
Clarksdale

SPAGHETTI AND MEATBALLS

SAUCE:
YIELD: 1 GALLON

1½ cups chopped onions
3 cloves garlic, chopped fine
⅓ cup chopped parsley
1½ cups chopped celery
½ cup bell pepper, chopped
2 to 3 tablespoons olive oil
3 pounds ground round or
ground chuck

6 (6 ounce) cans tomato paste
3 (6 ounce) cans water for
each can tomato paste
1 (6 ounce) can tomato juice
1 to 2 teaspoons Italian
seasoning (or to taste)
Salt and pepper to taste

In heavy 1½ gallon pot sauté vegetables in olive oil until soft, not brown. Add meat and cook until lightly browned. Add tomato paste, water, and tomato juice. Add seasonings. Simmer 2 to 2½ hours in heavy covered pot.

ITALIAN MEATBALLS:
SERVES: 8 TO 10

3 pounds ground chuck or
ground round
⅓ cup chopped parsley
2 stalks celery, chopped
½ cup chopped onions
3 garlic cloves, finely
chopped

⅓ cup chopped bell pepper
4 to 5 slices day-old bread,
crumbled
½ cup Romano or Parmesan
cheese
3 to 4 eggs
Salt and pepper to taste

Use processor to cut vegetables. Mix meat, vegetables, cheese, beaten eggs, and bread together. Add seasoning and mix well. Form meatballs the size of a small egg. Brown in skillet in oil. These may be frozen or refrigerated and added later to meat sauce. Let simmer 20 to 30 minutes in meat sauce.

Regina Youngblood
Lyon

Health Secret: To guard against food spoilage, thaw frozen meat or poultry in the refrigerator - not on the kitchen counter.

TORTELLINI

YIELD : 500 TO 600 2 INCH TORTELLINI

MEAT MIXTURE:

2½ pounds of ground chuck
   or ground round
½ pound pork sausage
1 wedge (4 ounce) Romano
   cheese, grated

8 large eggs
5 cloves garlic, chopped fine
3½ teaspoons nutmeg

Mix all ingredients well and set aside.

DOUGH:

12 eggs

7 cups plain flour

Mix eggs and flour well to form a soft dough. Knead well. Roll thin (about thickness of pie crust). Cut into two inch squares (or size desired). Place desired amount of meat mixture onto square, fold over and seal well with fork or pastry cutter. Cook covered in beef broth on medium heat for one hour or until dough is done. Uncooked tortellini may be quick frozen on a cookie sheet and then placed in freezer bags for use later. Do not need to thaw before cooking.

Carol Andrews
Clarksdale

VEGETABLE BEEF STEW

SERVES: 8 TO 10

1 pound beef, cubed
1 tablespoon oil
2 cups water
2 cups tomato juice
2 medium onions, chopped
1 (16 ounce) can whole
   tomatoes
1 (8¾ ounce) can corn,
   undrained

1 cup cubed potatoes
1 cup sliced carrots
1 cup chopped celery
1 cup green peas
1 cup lima beans
1 tablespoon sugar
2 teaspoons salt
2 teaspoons pepper
1 teaspoon hot sauce

In a large pot, brown beef in oil. Add all ingredients and bring to a boil. Reduce heat and cook for 2 hours.

Sherry M. Eason
Mattson

MEAT AND POTATO CASSEROLE

SERVES: 6 TO 8   OVEN: 350°

1 pound ground beef
1 onion, chopped
½ cup chopped celery
½ cup chopped pepper
1 (4 ounce) can drained
  mushrooms (optional)
1 tablespoon sugar added to
  meat mixture

Salt and pepper to taste
4 sliced potatoes
1 (10½ ounce) can tomato
  soup
1 cup grated cheese

Brown onion, celery, bell pepper and meat and mix together with mushrooms. Add sugar, salt and pepper. In a casserole put layer of potatoes, layer of meat mixture, sprinkle with cheese. Continue layering potatoes and meat in casserole. Mix tomato soup with one-half can water and pour over casserole. Bake forty-five minutes. Just before you take it out, add cheese on top and let it melt.

Family Secret: Men love this dish! For dieters or heart patients: use ground turkey instead of ground meat and use low salt or sodium tomato soup. Use low fat cheese and add one package of sugar substitute.

Mrs. M. D. Dunn, Sr., Mrs. Frank Wylie
Duncan

PEPPER STEAK

SERVES: 6

1 pound lean boneless
  sirloin steak, trimmed
1 tablespoon vegetable oil
1 clove garlic, peeled and
  crushed
½ to 1 teaspoon salt
1 teaspoon ground ginger
½ to 1 teaspoon pepper

2 large green peppers, cut in
  strips
2 large onions, thinly sliced
2 to 4 tablespoons soy sauce
½ teaspoon sugar
¾ cup beef broth
1 tablespoon cornstarch
¼ cup cold water

Freeze steak for about 1 hour to make it easier to slice. Cut slices ⅛ inch thick across the grain. Heat oil in large skillet. Add garlic, salt, pepper and ginger. Sauté just until garlic is slightly brown. Add steak slices. Brown lightly for 2 minutes; remove meat. Add green pepper and onion to same pan. Cook for 3 minutes. Dissolve cornstarch in cold water. Return beef to pan; add soy sauce, sugar, broth, and cornstarch dissolved in water. Simmer about 2 minutes until sauce thickens. Serve over hot cooked rice.

Emily Cooper
Clarksdale

RAVIOLI

YIELD: 50 DOZEN

STUFATO:

6 garlic buds
3 pounds rump roast
3 inch square salt meat
Small piece beef fat
1 large onion
1 cup red wine

1 cup chicken broth
Pinch of rosemary
Pinch of clove
Pinch of cinnamon
Bay leaf

Put garlic buds inside rump roast. Brown meat in small amount of margarine. Remove. Chop in food processor: salt meat, beef fat, and onion. Brown meats and add onion. Stir until softened. Add remaining ingredients and simmer for 30 minutes. Roast meat in this mixture in oven at 350° for 1 hour or until done.

STUFFING:

1 (10 ounce) package
  chopped spinach
2 large onions
¼ bunch parsley (stems
  removed)
3 celery ribs
2 to 3 carrots

The rump roast from Stufato
1 cup breadcrumbs
2 cups grated Parmesan
  cheese
12 eggs, more or less
Salt, pepper, nutmeg to taste
Broth if needed

Prepare spinach and drain well. Chop next 5 ingredients in food processor. Add next 3 ingredients and mix well. Add salt, pepper, and nutmeg. Add broth if too thick. Place stuffing by teaspoon fulls about 1½ inches apart on single sheet of pasta (see page 126); cover with second sheet. Seal and cut with crimper. Boil squares in undiluted chicken broth. Editor's note: I found it easier to make ravioli using ravioli pan. Follow directions accompanying the pan. Be sure to flour pan before each use.

SAUCE:

Stufato in which meat roasted
1½ (6 ounce) cans tomato
  paste

1 (28 ounce) can tomatoes
Grated Parmesan cheese

Add tomato paste and tomatoes to the stufato in which meat was roasted. Simmer for 30 to 45 minutes. When you put sauce on cooked ravioli, sprinkle freshly grated Parmesan cheese on top.

CONTINUED, RAVIOLI:

Family Secret: The stages of ravioli making are 4: The stufato (roasting the meat in seasoned liquids), the stuffing, the pasta, and the sauce. Do not try to make at one time. It is exhausting. Freeze stuffing in 1 pint containers omitting the eggs. Add 1 to 2 eggs to each pint after thawing. Freeze sauce in ½ pint containers. Should have 6 of each. Freeze completed ravioli on tray first and then put in packages so they won't stick together.

Perian Conerly
Clarksdale

LASAGNA

SERVES: 6 TO 8   OVEN: 350°

2 tablespoons salad oil
½ cup chopped onion
1 pound ground meat
1 teaspoon garlic powder
1 teaspoon salt
¼ teaspoon pepper
3 tablespoons parsley flakes
1 (10¾ ounce) can of tomato
   soup
18 ounce can tomato sauce
½ (1 pound) box lasagna
   noodles

½ cup grated Parmesan
   cheese
16 ounces grated mozzarella
   cheese
1 (16 ounce) carton cottage
   cheese
2 eggs, beaten
2 tablespoons parsley flakes
Salt and pepper to taste

Sauté onions in oil. Add meat and cook until red is gone. Add garlic powder. Add salt, pepper and parsley. Simmer 1 minute. Add soup and sauce. Simmer while you cook the noodles. Cook noodles according to package directions; drain. Mix Parmesan, mozzarella and cottage cheese. Add eggs, parsley, salt and pepper. Using 3 quart casserole dish, begin by putting a little meat sauce on bottom. Cover with layer of noodles, add ½ of cheese mixture and continue with layers, ending with sauce on top. Sprinkle Parmesan cheese on top. Bake for 30 minutes.

Mrs. John Morris
Clarksdale

BEEF AND BEAN SUPREME

SERVES: 8 TO 10   OVEN: 350°

2 pounds lean ground beef
1 large onion, chopped
1 bell pepper, chopped
1 cup chopped celery
1 pound can red beans
1 pound can pork and beans
1 (10¾) ounce can tomato
  soup
1 (10 ounce) can tomatoes
  and green chilies

1 can (4 ounce) sliced
  mushrooms
1½ teaspoons salt
1 tablespoon Worcestershire
  sauce
1 bay leaf, crumbled
Dash of hot sauce
1 cup grated sharp Cheddar
  cheese

Cook ground beef in large skillet, with no added fat, until it loses red color. Take meat out with slotted spoon. Cook until soft (low heat and covered) onion, bell pepper, and celery. Add all other ingredients except cheese and mix. Put in 3 quart casserole dish and sprinkle with cheese. Cook for 1 hour.

Family Secret: Served over the Delta's own healthful long-grain rice, Bean Supreme, is full of high-fiber beans, low-fat ground meat, and fresh vegetables. Try on a cold winter night over a bed of hot, fluffy rice, with a tossed salad and garlic French bread. Delicious!

Shirley Easley
Clarksdale

CAULIFLOWER WITH BEEF

SERVES: 4

1½ teaspoons soy sauce,
  divided
1 teaspoon salt, divided
Dash granulated garlic
½ teaspoon wine
½ pound thinly sliced tender
  beef (about ⅛ inch thick)
3 tablespoons vegetable oil,
  divided

2 pounds washed cauli-
  flower-Break into flowerettes, slice stalks into ½
  inch lengths. Parboil 2
  minutes and drain. Rinse
  in cold water.
½ cup chicken broth
1 tablespoon cornstarch
1 tablespoon water

CONTINUED, CAULIFLOWER WITH BEEF:

In a mixing bowl, place ½ teaspoon soy sauce, ½ teaspoon salt, granulated garlic, wine and sliced beef. Marinate 5 minutes. In a preheated wok or large skillet, add ½ teaspoon salt and 2 tablespoons oil. Turn to high heat and add cauliflower. Stir-fry for 1 minute. Remove and place aside. In the same utensil, place 1 tablespoon oil. Turn to high heat and add marinated beef. Toss and brown rapidly about 1 minute; remove beef and place aside. In the same utensil, place cauliflower, 1 teaspoon soy sauce and chicken broth. Cover and cook for 5 minutes. Remove cover. Add pre-browned beef. Stir in cornstarch mixture (1 tablespoon cornstarch mixed with 1 tablespoon water). Toss and mix continuously making sure liquid ingredients are well blended with cornstarch paste. When gravy thickens sufficiently to lightly coat the cauliflower and beef (about 2 minutes), remove from heat and serve immediately with hot steamed rice.

Lucy Leung
Baltimore, Maryland

BROCCOLI WITH BEEF

½ pound beef strips
1 tablespoon soy sauce
1 teaspoon cooking sherry
1 bunch broccoli
3½ tablespoons oil, divided
1 teaspoon salt, divided

2 whole cloves garlic,
   divided
¼ cup chicken broth
½ tablespoon cornstarch
½ tablespoon water

Slice beef into thin strips, about 2 inches wide. Marinate beef with soy sauce and cooking sherry from 30 minutes to 1 hour. Trim fibers off broccoli stem and cut into diagonal slices, about 1 inch by ¼ inch. Slice each floweret into 2 or 3 pieces. Heat 1½ tablespoons oil and add ½ teaspoon salt and 1 clove garlic. Add beef and stir-fry a minute. Remove beef and garlic. Discard garlic. Heat 2 tablespoons oil and add ½ teaspoon salt and 1 clove garlic. Add broccoli and stir-fry about 2 minutes. Add ¼ cup chicken broth (or water). Cover and simmer 4 to 5 minutes, or until desired tenderness. Remove and discard garlic. Return cooked beef to pan and mix with broccoli. Make a gravy by mixing the cornstarch with water. Add to broccoli and beef and stir until gravy thickens. Serve with rice.

Family Secrets: Same recipe may be used with other vegetables, such as bok choy, asparagus, bell pepper, cauliflower or snow peas.

Susan Chow
Memphis, Tennessee

SHAYK MIHSHI
(EGGPLANT AND MEAT CASSEROLE)

Because meat is sometimes difficult to obtain in the Middle East, vegetables are frequently used in its stead. Shayk Mihshi is a one-dish meal that was adapted in that way.

SERVES: 15 TO 20   OVEN: 350°

2 pounds ground chuck
1 large onion
½ cup pine nuts or pecans
3 large eggplants

2 (14 ounce) cans tomatoes
⅓ cup of water
Salt and pepper to taste

Brown meat with onions and nuts. Drain fat. Add salt and pepper to taste to cooked mixture. Allow meat to cool as you peel and slice eggplant into ¼ inch thickness. Using a 10 x 13 inch pan or casserole dish, layer eggplant, meat and tomatoes. Cover the bottom of pan with a layer of eggplant, layer eggplant with meat, and top with tomatoes. Continue layering until all eggplant and meat are used. Pour remaining tomatoes and ⅓ cup of water over all layers. Can be frozen or refrigerated at this time. When ready to bake, cover pan with top or foil. Bake for approximately one hour. At this time, sprinkle with grated cheese of choice, if desired. Uncover pan and cook for 10 additional minutes.

Louise Chamoun
Clarksdale

SWISS STEAK

SERVES: 4

2 to 3 pounds round steak
2 tablespoons flour
2 to 3 tablespoons oil
1 medium onion sliced and
pulled apart in rings
1 teaspoon mustard powder
½ teaspoon chili powder

1 small bay leaf
2 teaspoons Worcestershire
sauce
1 teaspoon sugar
2 cups canned tomatoes and
juice

Combine flour, salt, pepper, and round steak. On top of stove, heat oil in a large skillet and brown meat. Mix rest of ingredients and pour over steak. Simmer, covered, for 1½ hours. You will probably have to add a little water while cooking as some of the liquid will evaporate. You can also add cubed potatoes and cook with the meat.

Sherry Eason
Clarksdale

GARTRUDE'S PORK ROAST

OVEN: 250°

Large pork shoulder (blade) roast, have butcher trim off excess fat. Place roast in roaster with a drip pan or an oven broiler pan. It will take about 6 hours to cook a 6 pound roast. (Use meat thermometer to be sure.) Baste the roast with sauce (Gartrude's sauce) every hour, turn roast once or twice during cooking time, meanwhile go about your business. Thirty minutes before the roast is done, light grill or build a charcoal fire, and let coals die down. Place roasts on grill 45 minutes. I add hickory chips to my charcoal. I use the remaining sauce, over the sliced or chopped pork.

GARTRUDE'S BASTING SAUCE:
YIELD: 1 QUART

3 cups apple cider vinegar
10 tablespoons brown sugar
2 tablespoons salt
1 tablespoons black or white
   pepper
2½ teaspoons liquid smoke
1½ teaspoons red pepper

5 buttons garlic, crushed
1 medium onion, chopped
1 tablespoon chili powder
2 tablespoons water
1½ tablespoons cornstarch
2 sliced lemons

Mix first 9 ingredients in heavy pan. I use a 2 - quart Dutch oven. Bring to boil. Let simmer 30 minutes. Then add sliced lemons and cool. Store in quart jar in refrigerator. Keeps for months.

Hazel Boyd
Clarksdale

Health Secret: Animal fats are generally more saturated than vegetable fats.

CHINESE EGG ROLLS

YIELDS: 16 TO 20

1 small head of cabbage
1 bunch green onions
4 stalks celery
½ pound fresh bean sprouts
or 1 (14 ounce) can
1 pound lean, cooked pork,
ham or chicken

1 tablespoon chopped ginger
root
1 teaspoon garlic powder
2 tablespoons soy sauce
1 tablespoon corn starch
dissolved in ¼ cup water
1 pound package egg roll
wraps

Thinly slice cabbage, tops and bottoms of onions and celery. Put vegetables (including fresh bean sprouts) in large pan of boiling water (3 inches deep). Cook 5 minutes or until tender. Drain in colander rinsing with cold water. Drain canned bean sprouts, if used. Using an old kitchen towel, wring 1 cup batches of vegetables almost dry. Put vegetables in large mixing bowl and put aside. Cut meat into small pieces. Add to vegetables. Add ginger, garlic powder and soy sauce. Mix vegetables, meat and seasonings well. It's easiest to use your hands. Now you are ready to fill the wraps. Put 1 wrap in a diamond shape on counter in front of you, with corner pointing toward you. Put ¼ cup meat-vegetable filling horizontally about 1 inch below center of wrap. Fold corner nearest you over the filling. Bring left corner over, then right corner. Press the filling in securely. Using finger, spread dissolved cornstarch on the upper edges of remaining corner. Fold over like an envelope flap and press gently with fingers to seal. The finished roll will resemble a sealed package. Continue filling wraps until filling is gone. Egg rolls can be placed on a wax-paper lined cookie sheet and held for several hours before frying. Cover with plastic wrap to prevent drying. To fry egg rolls, heat 4 cups peanut oil in heavy skillet or wok over medium - high heat to about 375°. Fry 3 to 4 rolls at a time only until the pastry is golden on both sides. Place the fried rolls on end in a colander to drain off oil and then in a single layer on cookie sheet or plate lined with paper towels. Put in warm oven while preparing rest of meal or reheat briefly in microwave oven on high power. Serve with sweet sauce.

SWEET SAUCE:
6 ounces apricot preserves
⅛ to ¼ teaspoon cayenne
pepper
1 teaspoon chopped ginger
root

1 cup water
¼ teaspoon garlic powder

CONTINUED, SWEET SAUCE:

Combine all ingredients in saucepan. Heat to simmer, stirring to break up preserves. Simmer 10 to 15 minutes or until thickened to desired consistency.

Emily Cooper
Clarksdale

SZECHUAN PORK SHREDS AND BELL PEPPER

SERVES: 2 TO 3

8 ounce pork fillet
  (tenderloin)
1 large or 2 small red
  peppers
1 (3 ounce) can bamboo
  shoots

6 garlic cloves
4 slices fresh ginger
2 tablespoons cornstarch
Pinch of salt
3 tablespoons vegetable oil

Slice pork into paper thin slices, cutting across the grain, then stack the slices into piles of 5 or 6; cut into match stick shreds and set aside. (Easier to cut if slightly frozen.) Cut the peppers in half, trim and cut lengthwise into narrow shreds. Cut the bamboo shoots, garlic and ginger into similar pieces. Stir the cornstarch to coat the pork shreds, coating them evenly. Heat a wok over moderate heat and stir - fry the pepper shreds without oil until browned on the edges and half tender. Add a large pinch of salt, stir, then remove from wok. Add the oil and stir - fry the pork over high heat until pork turns white. Add the bamboo, garlic, and ginger and stir- fry for another minute; then add the pre - mixed seasoning sauce ingredients and return the pepper to the wok. Simmer, stirring, until the sauce thickens and clears; then serve with rice.

SEASONING SAUCE:
⅔ cup chicken broth
1 tablespoon light soy sauce
2 teaspoons wine or dry
  sherry

1 teaspoon cornstarch
½ teaspoon salt
Pinch of white pepper

Family Secret: For those who like it HOT!

Mamie Pang
Marks

PAN-FRIED EGG FOO YUNG

SERVES: ABOUT 8

6 eggs
¾ teaspoon salt
1 cup cooked meat or
  seafood*
1 cup fresh bean sprouts
  (washed)

½ cup diced celery
½ cup frozen peas (cooked)
¼ cup diced onion
2 tablespoons oil

*Crab, shrimp, roast pork, bacon, or ham...or combination Beat eggs; then season with salt. Shread or dice meat. Mix well with eggs. Add vegetables. Heat oil and spoon 2 to 3 tablespoons of egg mixture into pan to make one small omelet. (Fry each omelet separately.) Turn it over when bottom is done and brown lightly on the other side. Remove omelet and keep warm. Repeat process, adding more oil as needed. Serve omelets either plain, or with Egg Foo Yung sauce.

SAUCE:
¾ cup chicken broth
½ teaspoon salt
1 teaspoon soy sauce

2 tablespoons water
2 teaspoons cornstarch

Heat broth and stir in salt and soy sauce. Meanwhile blend cornstarch and cold water to a paste. Stir into broth to thicken. Spoon sauce over each omelet; or serve hot in a side dish as a dip.

Joanne Pang
Houston,Texas

SHISH-KA-BOB

SERVES: 4

1½ pounds sirloin steak
¼ cup mustard
¼ cup red wine vinegar
1 cup oil

¾ cup soy sauce
½ cup lemon juice
¼ cup Worcestershire sauce
1 tablespoon pepper

Cut beef into 1½ inch cubes. Combine next seven ingredients; pour over beef and marinate in refrigerator at least three hours. At cooking time thread marinated meat on skewers and broil or grill to desired degree or doneness. Brush with marinade while cooking.

Rita Moser
Clarksdale

PORK CHOPS WITH VEGETABLES

SERVES 6   OVEN: 350°

6 to 8 center cut pork chops
6 to 8 medium potatoes,
  peeled and sliced thin
1 (16 ounce) can English
  peas, drained
1 (16 ounce) can carrots,
  drained

Salt and pepper to taste
1 (10¾ ounce) can cream of
  onion soup
1 (10¾ ounce) cream of
  celery soup

Place pork chops in bottom of 9 x 13 inch pan. Layer thinly sliced potatoes, peas, and carrots alternately until all are used. Add salt and pepper to taste. Pour both cans of soup over mixture. Cover with foil and bake in preheated oven for 1 hour. Remove foil and bake for another 10 minutes.

Family Secret: Freezes well before baking.

Donna Davenport
Clarksdale

PORK CHOP CASSEROLE

SERVES: 4 TO 6   OVEN: 375°

1 cup uncooked rice
1 (4 ounce) can sliced
  mushrooms (optional)
2 tablespoons margarine
4 to 6 pork chops

Salt and pepper
1 small onion (sliced)
1 green pepper (sliced)
1 (10½ ounce) can beef
  bouillon

Preheat oven. Place uncooked rice, mushrooms and butter in a large glass casserole dish. Brown pork chops then season with salt and pepper; place on top of rice. On top of each chop, place a slice of onion and green pepper. Pour bouillon over all. Bake in tightly covered casserole for approximately 1 hour.

Family Secret: Serve with a vegetable and salad.

Carolyn Stringer
Clarksdale

Sherry Eason
Mattson, Mississippi

SMOKED BOSTON BUTT
WITH BAR - B - Q SAUCE

Over the years my husband, Philip, and I have entered barbeque cooking contests throughout the Mid-South. We treasure the friendships we have made while sharing recipes and cooking secrets with other barbecue teams.

SERVES: ABOUT ½ POUND PER PERSON   OVEN: 275°

Pork - Boston Butt 8 to 10
   pounds each

DRY RUBBING POWDER:
YIELD: 1¼ CUPS

6 tablespoons paprika	2 tablespoons red pepper
3 tablespoons onion salt	1 tablespoon black pepper
2 tablespoons garlic salt	1 tablespoon monosodium
2 tablespoons ground basil	glutamate
3 tablespoons dry mustard	

Mix all ingredients together and "rub" on pork butts before cooking

BAR - B - QUE SAUCE:
YIELD: APPROXIMATELY 1 GALLON

1 cup diced onions	½ pound dark brown sugar
½ cup margarine	3 tablespoons chili powder
3 bottles (28 ounces each)	¾ cup ketchup
hickory flavored BBQ	2 to 3 tablespoons hot sauce
sauce	3 tablespoons lemon juice
1 pound dark honey	

Simmer onions in melted margarine in a large cooking pot. Add remaining ingredients and simmer, stirring to blend in sugar. Simmer uncovered for 30 minutes. Let cool and refrigerate. This sauce is best when made one week before use, as spices have time to penetrate.

COOKING THE PORK BUTTS:
We use a large commercial cooker however, this will work with a small smoker. Prepare smoker accordingly. We use hickory wood and water smoker. Rub pork butts with dry rub then place meat in paper grocery sack and seal or roll sack up. Place meat on smoker

CONTINTUED, SMOKED BOSTON BUTT WITH BAR-B-Q SAUCE:

rack fat side down. Smoker should be kept on approximately 275° for 10 to 12 hours, depending of type of cooker and even cooking temperature. Two hours before serving, take meat out of sacks and place directly on rack to allow extra smoking time. Bone should twist out of meat and you will be able to tear meat or chop with ease. DO NOT SAUCE MEAT WHILE COOKING. SAUCE ONLY WHEN READY TO EAT. For a smaller crowd use a 4 to 6 pound Boston Butt. Rub with ⅓ to ½ cup dry powder. Follow cooking instructions as for large roast.

Family Secret: Serve with French bread, potato salad, barbecue beans, homemade orange sherbet or ice cream and iced tea. It is so good!

Nancy Daughdrill
Clarksdale

PORK TENDERLOIN WITH BARBEQUE SAUCE

SERVES: 8 TO 10   OVEN: 275°

4 to 5 pound pork tenderloin	2 tablespoons Worcestershire
1 tablespoon celery salt	sauce
1 teaspoon garlic powder	2 teaspoons coarse pepper
1 teaspoon onion salt	2 tablespoons liquid smoke
1½ teaspoons salt	1 teaspoon lemon juice

Combine marinade ingredients. Put tenderloin and marinade in large zip baggie; marinate meat in refrigerator for at least 12 hours. Transfer meat to roaster with top. Bake covered for 3 hours. Cool. Slice. Pour half the barbeque sauce over the meat and heat just before serving. Serve meat with rest of sauce in a bowl on the side.

BARBEQUE SAUCE:

½ cup catsup	½ onion, finely chopped
¼ cup wine vinegar	2 tablespoons lemon juice
Small jar baby food plums	1 teaspoon pepper
½ cup brown sugar	

Mix ingredients and simmer for 7 minutes, stirring often.

Dinni Clark
Columbus

CAPPELLETTI

One summer in Florida I sat Weezie Malvezzi and May Bolgeo down and elicited some of my favorite old-country recipes in a feeble effort to keep the tradition going. Since Italian cooking varies not only from region to region and village to village, but from kitchen to kitchen, you will no doubt encounter minor dissent should other Italian types read this. Even Weezie and May disagreed on several trivial points.

FILLING:

About half the meat from a boiled fat 4 pound hen (save broth)
1½ pounds lean cured ham
1½ pounds lean pork that has been roasted with rosemary, bay leaf, cinnamon, cloves

2 cups grated Parmesan cheese
6 well beaten eggs (check while adding)

* Freezing tip: If freezing filling, omit eggs. Freeze in 1 pint containers. After thawing, add 1 or 2 eggs to each pint. Bake or cook meats and grind all together. Add cheese and eggs. If mixture seems too soft, reduce the number of eggs.

PASTA:

1¾ cups flour   4 eggs

All eggs are not the same size. The density of the flour also varies so more eggs may be needed. If consistency of dough is wrong, add more flour if too thin; add a bit of water if too powdery. Make a well in the flour and break eggs in the middle. Stir until stiff, then work with the hands until thoroughly mixed. Allow dough to rest, covered with a tea towel, for about 15 - 20 minutes. Pinch off golf ball size amount of dough. Put dots of olive oil on hands and rub on dough before putting in pasta machine. Put dough ball through pasta machine 3 times on # 1 and one time on each other setting to desired thinness. (May need to flour a bit if the dough sticks on machine.)
* Make pasta as follows: Cut circles with a shot glass or use special cappelletti cutter. Dot each circle with small amount of filling. Fold over. Seal edges. (Shape now resembles half moon or fried apple pie.) Twist and mash into hat shape. Boil caps in chicken broth about 15 minutes and serve as a main dish soup. Top with Parmesan cheese.

CONTINUED, CAPPELLETTI

Family Secret: This is a two session venture. We make the filling one day; pasta, the next. "Cappelletti" means "little hats".

Perian Conerly
Clarksdale

CREAMY HAM TOWERS

SERVES: 8

1 chicken bouillon cube
½ cup hot water
1½ cups milk
¼ cup butter or margarine
¼ cup all-purpose flour
½ cup (2 ounce) shredded processed American cheese
1 teaspoon prepared mustard
1 teaspoon Worcestershire sauce

2 cups cubed cooked ham
⅓ cup sliced, pitted, ripe olives
2 tablespoons chopped pimiento
2 tablespoons minced fresh parsley
8 frozen puff pastry patty shells, baked

Dissolve bouillon cube in hot water; stir in milk and set aside. Melt butter over low heat in heavy saucepan; blend in flour. Cook 1 minute, constantly stirring. Add bouillon mixture gradually and cook over medium heat, stirring constantly until thickened and bubbly. Add cheese, mustard, and Worcestershire and stir until cheese melts. Stir in ham, olives, pimiento, and parsley. Heat thoroughly. Spoon into patty shells.

Family Secret: For a colorful luncheon serve with tomato aspic, fresh fruit with honey-celery seed dressing and banana muffins.

Mrs. Walter W. Thompson
Clarksdale

Health Secret: Adding a little more onion and garlic to your favorite recipe may help prevent cancer.

SALSICCIA CON SPINACI
(ITALIAN SWEET SAUSAGE WITH SPINACH)

YIELD: 4 TO 6

5 or 6 Italian sausages	1 (10 ounce) package frozen
2 tablespoons olive oil	spinach, cooked according
1 medium onion, sliced	to package directions
1 garlic clove, chopped	3 tablespoons tomato paste

Boil sausages (covered with water) for about 20 minutes to render fat. Remove and dry off. Brown lightly in olive oil. Remove from skillet. Add sliced onion and garlic clove into same skillet. Sauté till soft but not brown. Meanwhile, prepare spinach according to package instructions. Return the sausage to skillet. Add spinach, liquid and all. Add tomato paste. Simmer at least 45 minutes (covered) adding more water if necessary.

Toni Malvezzi Hardin
Duncan

SAVORY SAUSAGE CASSEROLE

SERVES: 6 TO 8   OVEN: 350°

1 pound bulk pork sausage (get medium or high priced)	1 cup sliced celery
	2½ cups water
	1 tablespoon soy sauce or Worcestershire
1 cup uncooked rice	½ cup roasted halved or slivered blanched almonds
2 packages (2 ounce) dehydrated chicken noodle soup	
¼ cup finely chopped onion	

Break apart sausage and brown it in an ungreased skillet, pouring off fat as it accumulates. Remove from burner. Mix together sausage, rice, soup, onion and celery and place in a 2 quart casserole. Refrigerate. When ready to bake, mix soy sauce with water and add this with the almonds to casserole. Mix all gently. Cover and bake for 1 hour.

Mrs. Charles Clark (Grace)
Clarksdale

YOUVETSI (BAKED LAMB CHOPS)

SERVES: 6 TO 8   OVEN: 375°

3 pounds lamb shoulder or   1 teaspoon sugar (optional)
   lamb chops   2 cups rosamarina
1 large onion, chopped   Salt and pepper
2 cups hot water   Several dashes of garlic
½ stick cinnamon   powder
2 eight ounce cans tomato   6 cups boiling water
   sauce

Rub lamb chops with salt, pepper, and garlic powder. Place in roasting pan and bake until meat begins to brown. Lower heat to 350° and add onions, cinnamon, tomato sauce, 2 cups water and sugar. Cook covered until meat is tender. When meat is completely cooked, remove from pan and add boiling water and rosamarina and bake for 30 minutes or until rosamarina is cooked. Stir occasionally. Serve lamb with rosamarina sprinkled with grated Parmesan cheese.

Family Secret: Serve with a green tossed salad. Rosamarina is a small round pasta about twice the size of rice.

Alexandra Peters
Clarksdale

TONYA'S HERBED LEG OF LAMB

SERVES: ABOUT 8   OVEN: 350°

1 leg of lamb (about 5   ½ teaspoon marjoram leaves
   pounds)   ½ teaspoon thyme leaves
2 cloves of garlic, crushed   1 teaspoon rosemary leaves
2 tablespoons olive oil   1 teaspoon seasoned salt
1 tablespoon cider vinegar   Black pepper to taste
2 teaspoons Worcestershire
   sauce

Crush garlic, add to olive oil and rub over leg of lamb. Pour vinegar and Worcestershire sauce over lamb and then sprinkle all the seasonings on top. Cook uncovered for 2 hours. Lamb will be crusty on outside and medium on inside. Add water to the drippings to make au jus. Juice can be thickened, if desired.

Tonya T. Marley
Sumner

BUTTERFLIED LEG OF LAMB

SERVES: 10 TO 12

1 6 - 7 pound leg of lamb
1 clove crushed garlic
¾ cup olive oil
¼ cup red wine vinegar
½ cup chopped onion
2 teaspoons prepared dijon -
   style mustard
2 teaspoons salt

½ teaspoon oregano
½ teaspoon basil
½ teaspoon thyme
½ teaspoon crushed rosemary
⅛ teaspoon freshly ground
   black pepper
1 crushed bay leaf

Bone the lamb and lay it flat, making incisions on both sides so it will lay flat. Place in flat glass dish or enameled tray and pour marinade made from all ingredients over the lamb. Marinate covered overnight in refrigerator. The enameled lower part of the broiler pan works well. It should be turned at least once while marinating. Remove at least one hour before broiling. Charcoal fire must be hot or gas grill heated hot. Grill 10 minutes each side, basting when you turn it. Allow meat to rest in a preheated oven, about 300° to keep warm, for 15 minutes before slicing thinly to serve.

Family Secret: For those who like their lamb rare. Most people can't tell it from beef when prepared in this manner. Serve with roasted new potatoes and green salad.

Edwin Mullens
Lyon

CHICKEN ASPARAGUS ALMONDINE

SERVES: 10   OVEN: 350°

10 chicken breasts
3 (10½ ounce) cans cream of
   mushroom soup
3 (15 ounce) cans asparagus,
   drained

1 (2 ounce) can pimento
½ can slivered almonds
2 (6 ounce) cans French fried
   onions

Brown chicken breasts. Place in three quart oblong casserole dishes. Put asparagus over chicken and sprinkle with pimento. Mix soup together in a medium bowl to break up lumps and pour over chicken. Sprinkle with almonds. Bake on hour. Top with French fried onions. Put back in oven to heat onions.

Family Secret: Serve with new potatoes, green salad and hot rolls.

Mary Eva Presley
Clarksdale

CHICKEN-SHRIMP SUPREME

SERVES: 10   OVEN: 350°

2 cups cut up, cooked
  chicken
2 cups cooked shrimp (crab
  boil, salt, and pepper to
  season water)
¼ cup butter (½ stick)
½ pound sliced mushrooms
  (2 cans)
2 tablespoons sliced, green
  onions

2 cans cream of chicken soup
½ cup sherry
½ cup light cream
1 cup shredded, Cheddar
  cheese
2 tablespoons chopped
  parsley
Hot buttered rice

In 3 quart saucepan melt butter, add onions, and mushrooms. Sauté 5 minutes. Add soup; gradually stir in cream and sherry. Add cheese and beat until melted. Add chicken and shrimp. Add parsley at last minute. Serve hot over rice or put half layer rice in casserole. Cover with sauce. Heat until bubbly in oven.

Mrs. Joe Mitchell (Pat)
Clarksdale

CHICKEN SPAGHETTI

SERVES: 8 TO 10   OVEN: 350°

3 to 4 pound hen, cooked
1 medium bunch celery
2 medium green peppers
2 small onions
1 tablespoon vegetable oil
1 (4 ounce) can mushroom
  pieces

2 (10¾ ounce) cans of cream
  of chicken soup
10 ounces sharp cheese, grated
9 ounces thin spaghetti,
  cooked and drained
Butter bread crumbs
Bacon chips

Remove hen from bones. Chop into bite-sized pieces. Chop celery, green pepper and onions. Sauté in vegetable oil until tender. Add soups and mushrooms. Stir to combine. Add cheese. Stir until melted. Add chicken; stir. Pour over cooked spaghetti. Mix thoroughly. Pour into greased 8 x 12 inch oblong casserole dish. Cover with bread crumbs and bacon chips. Bake uncovered for 1 hour.

Elsie Milligan
Clarksdale

CHICKEN ALBERGHETTI

Anna Maria Alberghetti, the beautiful vocalist from Pesano, Italy, used this recipe frequently because she could cook it ahead of time and reheat it later when the guests arrived.

SERVES: 6 TO 8   OVEN: 300°

4 whole chicken breasts, halved, skinned, boned
2 eggs, beaten
Fresh bread crumbs
Butter and olive oil, as needed
10½ ounces cream of mushroom soup

½ cup milk or half and half
8 slices Swiss cheese, paper thin
8 slices mozzarella cheese, paper thin
½ cup freshly grated Parmesan cheese
Butter

Dip chicken breasts halves in eggs. Roll in bread crumbs to coat all over. Fry chicken in half butter and half olive oil (butter burns too easily when used alone). Dilute cream of mushroom soup with milk. Cover bottom of 6 x 12 x 2 inch baking dish with soup and milk. Layer chicken on top of soup and milk. Top with slices of Swiss and mozzarella cheese. Sprinkle Parmesan cheese over all and dot with butter. Bake covered for 30 minutes. Uncover and cook 10 to 15 minutes more.

Family Secret: Can be cooked a day or two ahead and reheated for serving. I suggest a combination salad, white wine, and a dessert of your choice and rolls.

Amerina Biagoli Mei
Shaw

ALMOND CHICKEN

SERVES: 3

½ teaspoon salt
3 tablespoons vegetable oil
1 cup uncooked chicken filets cut into 1 x 1 inch pieces
½ cup diced water chestnuts
½ cup diced bamboo shoots
½ cup diced celery

¼ cup diced button mushrooms
½ cup chicken broth
1 teaspoon soy sauce
Cornstarch paste (2 tablespoons cornstarch mixed with 2 tablespoons water)
Toasted almond slivers

CONTINUED, ALMOND CHICKEN:

In a preheated wok or skillet, place salt and oil. Bring oil to a sizzling point. Add chicken. At high heat, toss and turn chicken until almost done (about 5 minutes). Reduce to medium heat and add water chestnuts, bamboo shoots, celery, and mushrooms. Increase to high heat, toss and turn until all ingredients are blended (about 3 minutes). Add chicken broth and soy sauce. Cover and cook at medium high heat for 5 minutes. Uncover. Gradually add cornstarch paste, stirring constantly. Continue to cook at medium high heat turning rapidly until liquids thicken and mixture is very hot (about 3 minutes). Garnish generously with almonds. Serve with hot steamed rice.

Shaw Pang
Clarksdale

SWEET AND SOUR CHICKEN WINGS

SERVES: 6

12 large chicken wings,   ¼ cup flour
   separated at joint   ¼ teaspoon salt
2 beaten eggs   ¼ teaspoon pepper
½ cup cornstarch   Oil for frying

Clean and dry chicken wings. Dip in eggs. In a large heavy paper bag place cornstarch, flour, salt and pepper. Drop egg coated chicken wings into bag, shake until completely coated. Deep fry chicken wings until golden brown. Drain on absorbent paper towels. Serve with sweet and sour sauce.

SWEET AND SOUR SAUCE:
1 cup vinegar   5 drops hot sauce
1 tablespoon catsup   Cornstarch paste (mix 1
1 teaspoon soy sauce   teaspoon cornstarch and 1
1 cup sugar   teaspoon cold water)
Pinch of salt

Combine all ingredients in a saucepan. Cook at high heat to boiling point, then thicken with cornstarch paste until medium thick. Add color to sauce with ½ cup pineapple tidbits, ¼ cup halved maraschino cherries, and ¼ cup bell pepper slivers, slightly steamed.

Sally Chow
Clarksdale

CHICKEN DELIGHTS

SERVES: 6

2 pounds boned chicken pieces	⅛ teaspoon ground pepper
½ cup bread crumbs	1 teaspoon oregano
½ cup Parmesan cheese	2 beaten eggs
1 teaspoon salt	1 cup white wine
	¾ cup salad oil

Pound chicken until thin. Pat dry and cut into pieces. Combine bread crumbs, Parmesan cheese, spices and salt. Set aside. Beat eggs in a shallow dish. Dip chicken into egg, then the crumb mixture, coating both sides. Heat oil in skillet. Sauté chicken until brown - about 3 minutes each side. Remove to warm platter. Drain fat, stir in wine. Scraping up brown residue until boiling. Pour over chicken.

Sue Bell
Clarksdale

CHICKEN AL POTAQUO

I can just picture my mother's Marcheganni relatives in Serra San Quirico Ancona, Italy every time I prepare this recipe.

SERVES: 4 TO 6

3 tablespoons vegetable oil	½ cup water (more if needed)
1 small onion, chopped	¾ cup vinegar
1 teaspoon dried parsley	¼ cup white wine (or water)
1 teaspoon black pepper	2½ to 3 pound chicken, cut up
1½ teaspoons salt	More salt and pepper to taste
2 small garlic cloves, minced	

Place oil, onion, parsley, salt and black pepper in a large heavy skillet or 11-inch electric skillet. Sauté slowly until almost brown; add garlic and cook until golden brown. Add chicken that has been sprinkled with salt and pepper and brown on all sides. Add vinegar and wine. Stir together. Let boil: cover and turn to simmer for 40 to 50 minutes. Add water when needed. Do not let it burn or become too dry.

Theresa Malatesta
Shaw

BARRISTERS' CHICKEN

SERVES: 4   OVEN 325°

4 chicken breasts, deboned   8 sticks ham
½ teaspoon salt   8 sticks Swiss cheese
1 to 5 teaspoons lemon   1 cup flour
   pepper

SAUCE:
1½ tablespoons butter   Salt and pepper to taste
½ cup zesty Italian dressing   8 ounce can of mushrooms

Pound chicken breasts flat. Wash and then sprinkle them with salt
and lemon pepper. Place ham and cheese on edge of chicken breast
and roll. Close with toothpicks. Repeat procedure always placing 2
sticks of ham and 2 sticks of cheese per chicken breasts. Dredge
breast with flour (season flour with lemon pepper and salt); sauté in
sauce in frying pan until brown. Remove, add mushrooms to top,
bake for 10 to 15 minutes.

W. Kurt Henke
Clarksdale

CHICKEN WITH PINE NUTS AND RICE

SERVES: 8   OVEN 350°

1 whole 3 - pound fryer or 8   2 cups rice
   chicken breasts   1 teaspoon salt
Salt for chicken   1 teaspoon black pepper
1 pound ground lamb, beef,   ½ teaspoon cinnamon
   or chuck   2 cups chicken broth
¼ cup pine nuts
2 tablespoons butter
   (preferably rendered)

Clean and cut fryer, season with salt and set aside. Brown meat:
drain. Brown pine nuts in butter; add pine nuts, rice, and seasonings
to meat. Mix thoroughly. Put meat and rice mixture in bottom of 11
x 14 inch pan. Place chicken on top. Pour broth over chicken and
rice. Bake for 45 to 50 minutes until chicken and rice are done.

Yvonne Rossie Abraham
Clarksdale

CHICKEN CROQUETTES
WITH GREEN PEAS IN CREAM SAUCE

SERVES: 4   OVEN: 365°

CROQUETTES:
3 tablespoons butter
¼ cup all-purpose flour
½ cup milk
½ cup chicken broth
1 tablespoon minced parsley
1 teaspoon lemon juice
1 teaspoon grated onion
Dash each of paprika and
    black pepper

1½ cups finely diced cooked
    chicken
¼ teaspoon salt
¾ cup fine dry bread crumbs
1 beaten egg
2 tablespoons water

Melt butter; blend in flour; add milk and broth. Cook and stir until mixture bubbles; cook and stir one minute longer. Add parsley, lemon juice, onion, and seasonings. Cool. Chop chicken very fine in food processor. Add chicken and salt to cream mixture and mix well. Chill. With wet hands, shape chicken mixture into eight balls, ¼ cup each (lightly packed). Roll in crumbs. Shape balls into cones; handling lightly so crumbs remain on outside. Dip into mixture of egg and water; roll in crumbs again. Fry in deep hot fat (365°) two to three minutes or until golden brown and hot through. Drain on paper towels; serve with green peas in cream sauce.

SAUCE:
2 tablespoons margarine
2 tablespoons flour
½ cup light cream
½ cup chicken broth

¼ teaspoon salt
½ cup drained, cooked
    English peas
Dash pepper

Melt butter; blend in all-purpose flour then add light cream and chicken broth all at once. Cook and stir until mixture thickens and bubbles. Add salt, dash pepper, and drained cooked or canned English peas (small ones). Heat through. Spoon over croquettes just before serving.

Mrs. Gus Brown, Jr.
Marks

OVEN-FRIED SESAME CHICKEN

SERVES: 4   OVEN: 400°

2 tablespoons soy sauce   ¼ teaspoon salt
2 tablespoons flour   4 skinned chicken breasts
2 tablespoons sesame seed   2 tablespoons melted butter

In shallow dish place soy sauce and coat each piece of chicken well. Mix next three ingredients on a piece of waxed paper. Dip chicken in flour mixture (on flesh side only) and arrange with that side up in a 9 x 13 inch pan. Drizzle melted butter over. Bake 40 minutes or until tender.

Mrs. Hartley Kittle
Clarksdale

CHICKEN CURRY

SERVES: 10

1 (5 pound) hen   3 tablespoons Worcestershire
1 large onion   sauce
1 cup celery with leaves   4 tablespoons flour
½ pound bacon   ½ cup cold water
2 large onions, chopped   Salt and pepper to taste
8 stalks celery, chopped   2 egg yolks
4 apples   1 cup half and half cream
3 tablespoons curry powder   5 cups rice
1 teaspoon ginger

Cook hen in 2 quarts water with celery and onion. Remove in slivers, let broth cool, skim fat. In skillet, fry bacon until crisp, add the two onions and celery; and peeled and chopped apples. Add curry powder, ginger, Worcestershire. Cook 5 minutes. Add the 2 quarts stock. Blend 4 tablespoons flour in ½ cup cold water. Add to mixture, stirring to thicken. Add salt and pepper to taste. Add chicken. Let sit over night in refrigerator or several hours to develop flavor. To reheat, place over hot water, add beaten yolks and half and half.

CONDIMENTS:
Chutney   Stuffed olives, chopped
½ pound bacon, fried and   Grated coconut
   crumbled   Toasted sliced almonds

Serve over rice, using the condiments listed above.

Mrs. Harris Barnes, Jr.

KATIE'S CHICKEN CASSEROLE

SERVES: 10 TO 12   OVEN: 350°

3 cups cooked chicken (cut into bite size pieces)
1 tablespoon lemon juice
1 package seasoned long grain and wild rice (cook according to package directions)
2 cans cream of celery soup
1 large jar chopped pimentos; drained

1½ cups mayonnaise
1 can French style green beans; drained or 1 can artichoke hearts; drained and sliced
1 can sliced water chestnuts; drained
Salt, pepper, garlic salt, and soy sauce to taste

Sprinkle chicken with lemon juice. Mix all ingredients and place in a 9 x 13 inch casserole.

TOPPING:
Small package slivered almonds
1 package seasoned bread stuffing

1 stick margarine

Melt margarine and mix stuffing crumbs. Top casserole with this mixture and sprinkle slivered almonds on top. Bake uncovered for 25 minutes or until thoroughly hot.

Mrs. Billy Frazer
Mrs. Stan Hayes
Clarksdale

FRESH ASPARAGUS CHICKEN WITH BLACK BEAN SAUCE

SERVES: 3 TO 4

1½ pounds fresh green asparagus, pared 1 inch below green part and sliced diagonally into ½ inch thick slices
2 cups boiling water
2 tablespoons vegetable oil
½ teaspoon salt
1 cup white meat of chicken cut in ¾ inch squares (uncooked)

1 tablespoon mashed fermented black beans, combined with 1 clove mashed garlic and 1 tablespoon soy sauce
¼ teaspoon sugar
½ cup chicken broth
1 tablespoon cornstarch
1 tablespoon water

CONTINUED, FRESH ASPARAGUS CHICKEN WITH BLACK BEAN SAUCE:

In a sauce pot, place boiling water and asparagus. Cook at high heat for 1 minute. Drain and rinse in cold water. In a preheated wok or skillet, place 2 tablespoons vegetable oil and salt. Increase to high heat and add sliced asparagus. Stir-fry for 1 minute. Remove from pan. Stir-fry chicken 2 to 3 minutes. Add black bean sauce mixture. Add sugar. Add asparagus and chicken broth. Toss and mix rapidly but gently for 2 minutes. Gradually add cornstarch mixture (1 tablespoon cornstarch and 1 tablespoon water). Continue to cook at high heat, turning and mixing constantly 1 to 2 minutes until sauce is just thick enough to coat asparagus and chicken. Remove from heat and serve with steamed rice.

Alfred Leung
Baltimore, Maryland

PINEAPPLE CHICKEN

SERVES: 4

4 chicken breasts cut into 1 x 1 inch pieces	Oil for frying
¾ teaspoon salt, divided	½ cup vinegar
1 egg	½ cup sugar
⅛ teaspoon granulated garlic	⅓ cup catsup
½ teaspoon soy sauce	4 drops hot sauce
⅛ teaspoon pepper	1 cup canned pineapple chunks
Cornstarch paste (1 tablespoon cornstarch mixed with 1 tablespoon water)	½ cup green pepper, sliced into 1 x 1 inch pieces

Mix together chicken, ½ teaspoon salt, egg, granulated garlic, soy sauce and pepper. Dust lightly and evenly with cornstarch. In a preheated wok or skillet, place 2 inches vegetable oil. Bring oil to sizzling point at high heat. Add chicken and deep fry until brown. Drain on absorbent paper towels. Drain oil from wok or skillet. Place vinegar, sugar, ¼ teaspoon salt, ⅓ cup catsup, and hot sauce in wok. Cook at medium heat to boiling point, then thicken with cornstarch paste until medium thick. Add pineapple, green pepper, and chicken. Toss and mix thoroughly until chicken is heated through. Serve immediately with hot steamed rice.

Walter Pang

FORTY CLOVE CHICKEN

SERVES: 4 TO 6   OVEN: 375°

1 fryer - cut in pieces
40 cloves fresh garlic
½ cup dry white wine
¼ cup dry vermouth
½ cup olive oil
4 stalks celery - cut in one
  inch pieces

1 teaspoon oregano
2 teaspoons dry basil
6 sprigs parsley, minced
Pinch red pepper
1 lemon
Salt and pepper to taste

Place chicken, skin side up, in shallow baking dish. Sprinkle all ingredients over the chicken. Squeeze juice from lemon on top. Cut remaining lemon into slices and arrange on top. Cover with foil. Bake for 40 minutes.

Family Secret: You will not believe it, but your kitchen will not smell like Italy. Please feel free to eat garlic. Delish!!

Johnnie Lubiani
Clarksdale

LOUISIANA CHICKEN & VEGETABLE SAUTÉ

SERVES: 2 TO 3

2 deboned, skinned chicken
  breasts
1 carrot
1 zucchini squash
1 yellow squash
2 celery stalks
1 small sliced onion

5 ounces butter or margarine
½ teaspoon sage
Salt and pepper to taste
Angel hair pasta or your
  favorite pasta
Grated Parmesan cheese

Cut chicken into strips. Cut julienne strips of carrot, zucchini squash, yellow squash and celery. Lightly brown chicken in butter then sauté vegetables on medium high heat stirring constantly until vegetables are tender. Add salt and pepper to taste and add sage. Toss gently and pour over cooked pasta. Sprinkle with grated Parmesan cheese and serve.

Carolyn Stringer
Clarksdale

MANDARIN ORANGE CHICKEN

YIELD: 4 TO 6   OVEN: 350°

4 to 6 chicken breasts, split
¼ teaspoon salt
¼ teaspoon pepper
¼ teaspoon monosodium
   glutamate
¼ cup margarine or butter
11 ounce can of mandarin
   oranges and juice

¼ cup soy sauce
1 tablespoon all-purpose
   flour
1 teaspoon prepared mustard
1 teaspoon vinegar
¼ teaspoon garlic powder
1 teaspoon minced onion
¼ cup pineapple preserves

First wipe chicken with wet paper towels; rub with ¼ teaspoon pepper and monosodium glutamate. Sauté chicken in margarine or butter until brown on both sides. Then remove chicken from margarine. Remove skins, if desired. Drain juice from orange slices, add soy sauce and flour to the juice. Stir until smooth, adding mustard, vinegar, garlic powder, onion, and pineapple preserves. Pour over chicken, which has been placed in casserole. Cover, cook 1 hour. Add oranges last 10 minutes of cooking time. Serve over rice.

Susan Connell
Clarksdale

GEORGIA'S CHICKEN POT PIE

SERVES: 6 TO 8   OVEN: 375°

1 (3 pound) fryer, boiled and
   cut into bite sized pieces
1 (10¾ ounce) can chicken or
   chicken mushroom soup
2 cups chicken broth
3 hard boiled eggs, cut up

1 (4 ounce) can drained
   mushrooms
1 cup self-rising flour
1 cup milk
½ cup melted butter (mixed
   and whisked)

Mix first 5 ingredients together and pour into a greased 2 quart round casserole. Mix flour, milk, and butter together and ladle carefully over top of chicken. Bake about 45 minutes to 1 hour or until brown.

Georgia Haaga
Clarksdale

GRAVES CHICKEN PASTA MEDLEY

SERVES: 8 TO 10

2 packages tri-color noodles	Mayonnaise
1 stick margarine	Buttermilk
6 medium squash	4 to 6 chicken breasts
6 carrots (peeled)	(skinned and boned),
1 bunch broccoli	coated lightly with Cajun
1 tablespoon Greek	seasoning
seasoning	
1 package buttermilk salad	
dressing mix	

Slice and dice squash and carrots. Add broccoli flowerettes. Place in sauté pan with 1 stick margarine and 1 tablespoon Greek seasoning. Sauté slowly while cooking noodles according to package instructions. Drain noodles, spray with cool tap water and toss with 1 tablespoon olive oil. Place pan under colander and pour sautéed vegetables over noodles. Let drain. Grill chicken breast until done. Cut and dice, and add chicken to vegetable/noodle mixture. Put in large pan and lightly toss with small amount of buttermilk salad mix: Mix according to package instructions except half the mayonnaise and double the buttermilk.

Barbara Graves
Clarksdale

STUFFED CHICKEN BREASTS SAVANNAH

SERVES: 8   OVEN 325°

4 whole chicken breasts,	1 cup dry white wine
skinned, boned and halved	¼ cup finely chopped onion
4 thin slices boiled ham, cut	½ teaspoon salt
in half	Pepper to taste
8 slices Swiss cheese	1 cup milk
½ cup all purpose flour,	1 cup half and half
divided	Chopped fresh parsley
1 egg, slightly beaten	Hot cooked rice or noodles
⅔ cup fine dry bread crumbs	
½ cup plus 2 tablespoons	
melted butter, divided	

142

CONTINUED, STUFFED CHICKEN BREASTS SAVANNAH:

Flatten chicken breasts with meat mallet. Place a slice of ham and cheese on each chicken breast and roll up and secure with wooden picks. Dredge each roll in ¼ cup of flour and dip in egg; coat well with bread crumbs. Lightly brown on all sides in ¼ cup butter. Add wine; simmer covered for 20 minutes. Remove rolls and place in a shallow baking dish, reserving drippings. Sauté onion in 6 tablespoons butter until tender, stirring occasionally. Blend in remaining ¼ cup flour, salt and pepper. Gradually add milk and half and half, stirring constantly until smooth and thickened. Pour sauce over rolls, bake uncovered for 20 minutes. Garnish with parsley. Serve over rice or noodles.

Sherry Eason
Mattson

ITALIAN STUFFED CHICKEN

In Italy many recipes developed from foods readily available from family farms and gardens. The Agostinelli's most often used day-old home-made bread for the stuffing in this dish.

SERVES: 6   OVEN: 350°

3 cups firmly packed grated
   French bread (day old)
¼ cup fresh parsley, chopped
¼ cup Parmesan cheese
½ teaspoon Italian seasoning
1 tablespoon lemon, grated
   (rind and meat)
1 teaspoon finely chopped
   garlic (maybe more to your
   taste)

3 large eggs, beaten
1 large chicken, 4 to 5
   pounds
Salt, pepper, and garlic salt to
   taste
2 tablespoons oil

Mix dry ingredients together. Add beaten eggs and mix. Add oil and water if needed to make soft consistency that will mold together. Stuff this in cavity of chicken. Pin or sew chicken to close cavity. Rub chicken with oil, salt, pepper, and garlic salt. Spray large roaster with cooking spray. Cook covered for 1 hour. Then remove cover and bake another hour. May need to add water for juice while cooking.

Family Secret: Can cook sweet potatoes, white potatoes, or carrots in pan with chicken. Can use rolled round steak instead of chicken. Cook at 250° for 2 to 2½ hours.

Regina A. Youngblood

BARBECUE CHICKEN

SERVES: 6   OVEN: 325°

1 chicken or pieces, with or
  without skin

COATING:
½ cup flour   1 teaspoon paprika
½ cup butter
2 teaspoons each of salt and
  pepper

SAUCE:
¾ cup water   1 tablespoon chopped
¾ cup catsup   parsley
2 tablespoons grated onion   Garlic to taste (very little-1 bud)

Dip chicken pieces in heated coating and place in shallow pan (13 x
9 x 2 inches). Heat sauce to boiling. Pour over chicken and bake 1
hour.

                                     Mrs. Lee Graves, Jr.
                                     Clarksdale

RUMAKI

SERVES: 2 TO 3

4 ounces chicken livers   ¾ teaspoon monosodium
1 small can sliced water   glutamate, divided
  chestnuts   2 cups self-rising flour
1½ teaspoons salt, divided   1 cup cornstarch
1 teaspoon soy sauce   Bacon
2 drops sesame oil   1 box wooden toothpicks

Boil chicken livers for 5 minutes or until done. Cut the liver the
same size as the water chestnut slices. Marinate liver with ½ teaspoon
salt, ¼ teaspoon monosodium glutamate, soy sauce, and sesame oil
for 30 minutes. Drain water chestnuts. In a shallow pan, combine
flour, cornstarch, 1 teaspoon salt and ½ teaspoon monosodium
glutamate. Mix thoroughly. Cut several strips of bacon in half.
Wrap bacon around 1 piece of liver with one piece of water chestnut.
Poke a toothpick through the water chestnuts and liver to secure
the bacon. Continue process until all chicken livers have been used.
Pat the fixed pieces firmly with the flour mixture. Fry in a deep
fryer for 3 minutes.

                                     Jean Wong
                                     Clarksdale

CHICKEN ON SKEWER

SERVES: 6 TO 8

24 pearl onions, peeled
6 boned, skinned chicken breasts, cut into one - inch strips
2 red, green, or yellow bell peppers, seeded and cut into 1 inch strips
¾ cup soy sauce
⅓ cup packed brown sugar
⅓ cup sherry
⅓ cup lemon juice
3 tablespoons creamy peanut butter
2 cloves garlic, minced
1½ tablespoons fresh ginger root, minced
Dash hot sauce

Place onions, chicken, and peppers in shallow non - metal container. For marinade, place remaining ingredients in blender or food processor; cover and blend. Pour mixture over chicken and vegetables. Cover. Chill at least one hour; preferably overnight. Stir mixture occasionally to distribute marinade. Drain marinade; reserve for basting. Pat chicken and vegetables, dry with paper towels. Thread chicken, onions, and peppers on eight skewers. Brush generously with marinade. Grill about three inches from hot coals, turning once, for 8 - 10 minutes or until chicken is done. Brush often with marinade while cooking. Serve hot.

Family Secret: Great with wild rice and spinach salad.

Emily Cooper
Clarksdale

CHICKEN AND SPINACH

SERVES: 6   OVEN: 350°

4 packages chopped spinach, cooked and drained
6 chicken breasts, deboned and skinned
Flour
Margarine
Salt, pepper, granulated garlic
2 cartons plain whipping cream
Parmesan cheese
Paprika

Cook and drain chopped spinach. Press into 9 x 13 inch well - greased pan. Dip chicken breasts in flour first and then melted margarine. Place over spinach. Season liberally with salt, pepper, and granulated garlic. Pour 2 cartons of plain whipping cream over casserole. Generously, sprinkle with Parmesan cheese. Can decorate with paprika. Bake uncovered for 1 hour.

Beverly Grant
Clarksdale

CREAMED TURKEY

SERVES: 4

2 cups of cooked turkey	1½ cups of whole milk
1 tablespoon of celery seed	Salt if needed
½ cup turkey broth	Toast points, buttered
1 tablespoon of cornstarch	

Cube turkey into small pieces. If you have no left over turkey slices, you can boil the carcass. You may use any amount of turkey, but adjust cream sauce amount accordingly. Boil turkey with celery seed and turkey broth for several minutes. Add cornstarch to ½ cup cold milk. Add remaining 1 cup of milk to turkey mixture and bring to a boil. Add a little of the hot mixture to the cornstarch mixture, then add to the turkey. Boil until thick and serve on toast points.

Family Secret: Good served with baked apples.

Eileen M. Casburn
Sumner

TURKEY BREAST

OVEN: 325°

Any size frozen turkey breast	Slices of onion
Butter	2 ribs of celery
Salt and pepper	Bottled brown bouquet sauce

Rinse frozen turkey breast and pat dry. Rub with softened butter and salt and pepper. In a large skillet, lined crossways with aluminum foil, place slices of onion and 2 stalks celery on bottom. Place frozen breast on this and close foil tightly. Cook for 1 hour per pound. Then turn oven to 450° and open foil to brown the meat. The broth can be used to make gravy with equal parts of butter, flour, and a few drops of bottled brown bouquet sauce to darken gravy. Unbelievably easy! And makes such a moist turkey!

Jane Longino
Clarksdale

TURKEY HASH (BEST PART OF THE TURKEY)

Turkey Hash is a must for the day after Thanksgiving at our house. I have a friend from Texas who never fails to call over the holiday and say, "Tell me one more time how to make Turkey Hash"!

SERVES: 8

Leftover turkey, bones and all	4 large potatoes, cubed
6 cups water, more or less	1 teaspoon salt
4 ribs celery, chop in ½ inch slices	1 tablespoon pepper
2 onions, chunk chopped	2 tablespoons Worcestershire sauce

Break turkey apart, breast section from leg section. Place in stock pot or a pot that holds at least 1 gallon liquid. Barely cover turkey with water. Simmer until all meat falls off bone. Remove bones, skim fat off. Add celery and onions. Let them cook for 15 minutes. Then add cubed raw potatoes. Simmer until potatoes are done. Add salt, pepper and Worcestershire.

Family Secret: Serve Turkey Hash over rice or toast with tossed salad.

Roselyn Dulaney
Clarksdale

ITALIAN BAKED TURKEY

OVEN: 350°

Wash any size turkey thoroughly and pat dry. Cover with butter or olive oil then pat Aline's Northern Italian Seasoning (page 70) all over turkey - under wings, legs and inside. Salt and pepper to taste. Put in roaster. Pour 1 cup wine (any kind) gently over turkey. Add 1 cup water to roaster. Cover; cook until done.

Family Secret: Every slice will be moist. You cannot use drippings in your dressing because of the wine flavor.

Aline Alias
Clarksdale

Health Secret: Bran cereal can be substituted for cracker or bread crumbs or potato chips in casseroles, meatloaf or as a coating for chicken or fish.

SMOTHERED ANTELOPE
(OR VENISON) STEAK

When my husband, Jim, began going to Wyoming in the fall to hunt antelope, it was up to me to devise a way to serve the meat he brought home. This recipe is the result of my testing.

SERVES: 16   OVEN: 275°

About 2½ pounds steak
Salt and pepper
1 tablespoon dry mustard
Flour
Bacon grease
1 (10¾ ounce) can consommé
1 tablespoon dried parsley
1 chicken bouillon cube

⅔ cup water
⅔ cup dry wine
2 bay leaves
6 juniper berries
1 large sliced onion
2 stalks julienne celery
1½ cups coarsely chopped
  carrots

Trim all fat and sliver skin from meat and cut in serving size pieces. Sprinkle with salt, pepper, and dry mustard. Pound in a little flour with the edge of a saucer. Brown on both sides in bacon drippings and remove from pan. Add to pan, ½ can consommé, parsley, bouillon cube, water, wine, bay leaves, juniper berries, and 1 tablespoon more flour. Bring to a good boil and return steak to pot. Cover meat with onion slices and julienne celery. Bake 2½ hours. Add carrot chunks for last hour if desired.

Family Secret: The gravy from this is good. I like mashed potatoes with the meat gravy and lettuce and tomato salad for a tart taste to accompany.

Nan M. Russell
Jonestown

VENISON SHISH KA BOBS

SERVES: 4 TO 6

2 pounds of deer tenderloin, cubed
1 small bottle Italian dressing

1 small bottle Worcestershire sauce

CONTINUED, VENISON SHISH KA BOBS

CUBE:

Potatoes	Bell pepper
Onions	Salad tomatoes
Whole mushrooms	

Marinate venison in dressing and sauce in covered dish in refrigerator overnight. Alternate meat and vegetables on skewers and cook on grill until done.

Mike Simpson
Clarksdale

PEALICKER PLANTATION DUCK GUMBO

The lands along the southern Mississippi River were and continue to be a wildlife haven. Teddy Roosevelt used to camp on what is now the front lawn of Pealicker Plantation. He and his entourage hunted bear, deer, turkey, duck and other game. This duck gumbo was perfected to feed present-day hunters who still flock to the area from far regions of the country.

SERVES: 10 TO 12   OVEN: 325°

4 ducks	6 stalks celery
1 chicken	1 (10 ounce) box frozen okra
10 tablespoons oil	(chopped)
12 tablespoons flour	1 large can tomatoes
10 cups broth from chicken	1 package crab boil
1 bell pepper, chopped	3 tablespoons gumbo filé
1 onion, chopped	Salt and pepper to taste

Bake ducks with small amount of water, covered, in oven 2 hours. Boil chicken in at least 10 cups of water. Reserve broth. Debone ducks and chicken and cut into bite size pieces. Heat oil in 10 quart pot, add flour stirring until smooth, remove from heat, add chicken broth. Return to heat. After bubbling, add chopped vegetables - pepper, onion, celery - cook until tender. Lower heat to simmer. Add tomatoes, okra, gumbo filé, salt and pepper. Mix well. Add bag of crab boil - do not stir. Simmer covered at least 2 hours.

Remove bag of crab boil after seasoned to your taste. Serve hot over rice.

Mrs. Jean Duff
Alligator

WILD DOVES OR QUAIL

SERVES: 4   OVEN: 350°

8 doves or quail   1 stick margarine
Salt   1 cup water
Pepper

Wash birds and dry them. Sprinkle with salt and pepper. Place in a
skillet containing melted margarine and brown on all sides. Turn
temperature to low or 3 on an electric range. Add 1 cup water if
doves get too dry. If you add too much water you must add
margarine. Cook at least 1½ hours. You cannot cook them too long.
Serve on salt rising toast. Buy the salt rising bread at a specialty
bakery and keep frozen.

Penny Frazer
Clarksdale

BAKED DOVE BREASTS ON TOAST POINTS

SERVES: 8 TO 10   OVEN 250°

18 to 20 dove breasts   1 cup consommé soup
Peanut oil   1 tablespoon Worcestershire
1 teaspoon salt   sauce
Fresh ground pepper   ½ cup dry sherry
Dry mustard, about 1   1 small chopped onion
   teaspoon

Wash and dry breasts well with paper towel. Put some peanut oil in
a shallow bowl and completely coat breasts in oil. Place in a Dutch
oven, breast side up and sprinkle on salt, pepper and dry mustard.
Combine consommé, sherry, Worcestershire sauce and chopped
onion and pour into Dutch oven with birds. Be careful and don't
wash off the oil or birds will cook dry. Bake 2 hours and if the
breasts aren't very tender, cook a bit longer. Cover your Dutch oven
so the birds don't get dry.

Family Secret: Serve the breasts on toast points and spoon some
sauce from the pan over them. I like a rice dish with this and a tart
fruit of some kind and a bland green vegetable (English peas are
nice). See my "Baked Pineapple and Cheese Casserole."

Nan M. Russell
Jonestown

WILD DUCKS IN WINE (STUFATO)

YIELD: 2 QUARTS

4 wild ducks, quartered	½ teaspoon allspice
¼ cup margarine or butter	3 or 4 cups inexpensive
1 pound ground beef, salted	Italian red wine
1 large onion, chopped fine	3 cups water (or more)
2 bay leaves	1 (14½ ounce) can tomatoes
1 teaspoon rosemary	broken into pieces
½ teaspoon cinnamon	½ (6 ounce) can tomato paste

Melt margarine in large pot. Lightly brown ducks. Remove ducks from pot. Salt and pepper ducks generously. Brown ground beef in pot. Stir in onion and cook till soft. Return ducks to pot along with the spices, wine, water, tomatoes, and tomato paste. Simmer slowly 4 hours or longer. Duck should be cooked until meat almost falls from bone and serve over polenta or Gnocchi (See below).

Family Secret: May use 4 squirrels or 4 small rabbits instead of ducks. Freezes well.

Toni Malvezzi Hardin
Duncan

GNOCCHI

SERVES: 2 TO 3

2 medium to large potatoes	1 to 2 tablespoons vegetable
1 to 1¼ cups flour	oil (not olive)

Boil potatoes in skins until done. Pull off skins. Put through ricer or cream in food processor. Flour clean counter top. Put potatoes on counter and gradually work in flour and oil with hands until it reaches a dough - like consistency. The amount of flour and oil may vary. Cut the dough into 3 to 4 pieces. Roll each piece out like a snake - about ½ inch by 16 to 18 inches. Cut each "snake" into ¾ inch sections. Roll each section over the tines of a fork, so it looks like a sea shell. Drop Gnocchi into boiling water and cook 2 to 3 minutes or until they come to top. Drain and serve with Stufato (page 151).

Toni Malvezzi Hardin
Duncan

DUCK GUMBO

We cook this in a 4 gallon and a 5 gallon pot. One time the only long handled spatula we had broke as Elzy was cooking. He decided a boat paddle was the best thing to use for stirring. Since then we have saved that paddle just for gumbo.

SERVES: 40 TO 50   OVEN: 350°

STEP ONE:

12 to 16 ducks   ½ ham (sliced)
1 small turkey or 2 to 3 hens
10 pounds smoked cured hot
   Italian sausage

Boil ducks and turkey (or hens) in water seasoned with:

8 or 10 sliced onions   3 or 4 bay leaves
10 or 12 sliced carrots   Salt, pepper, and Creole
2 bunches celery   seasoning
2 or 3 cloves garlic

Remove ducks and turkey, debone and chop. Strain stock and set aside to use later.

STEP 2:

Slice sausage. Brown ham and sausage in heavy skillet. Cut in bite size pieces to add to gumbo. Add water to skillet to remove brown particles. Add all of this to stock because it adds flavor.

STEP: 3

8 to 10 pounds fresh okra (sliced) frozen may be substituted. Fry okra until ropiness disappears — 30 minutes or more — stirring frequently to avoid burning. Set aside to add to gumbo.

STEP 4: ROUX (A DELICATE PROCEDURE)

2 cups flour   6 cloves garlic, minced fine
2½ cups cooking oil   or pressed
10 to 12 chopped onions   10 to 12 carrots, chopped (if
6 bell peppers, chopped   you like)
3 stalks or bunches of celery,
   chopped

CONTINUED, DUCK GUMBO

Mix flour and oil. Cook until dark brown. Remember never to cook too fast, and stir constantly. When it reaches that dark brown color, remove from fire immediately and add onions, bell peppers, celery, garlic, and carrots. Continue stirring until it cools down. Add hot stock, stirring as you go. Place back on fire and add rest of ingredients (ducks, turkey, ham, sausage, and okra). Add seasonings to taste — salt, pepper, red pepper, bay leaves, hot sauce, and Worcestershire. Add water to desired thickness. Simmer approximately two hours — serve over rice. Enjoy! ! !

Family Secret: We serve this with a tossed salad and good red wine, and cheese cake for dessert. Serve the gumbo over rice.

Mary and Elzy Smith
Lyon

DUCK STROGANOFF

SERVES: 10 TO 12   OVEN: 325°

4 wild ducks, parboiled; remove meat from bones and dice	1 large can sliced mushrooms
	1 teaspoon oregano
	1 teaspoon rosemary
2 medium onions, chopped and sautéed in butter	¼ cup chopped parsley
	2 teaspoons bottled brown bouquet sauce
1 can cream of mushroom soup	Salt and pepper, to taste
1 can cream of celery soup	2 cups sour cream

Place meat in large baking dish. Mix sautéed onions and other ingredients and pour over meat. Stir to mix. Cover and bake one hour, stirring occasionally. Add sour cream and mix well. Serve over wild rice of white and wild mix.

Family Secret: Good served with congealed orange-pineapple salad or with a tossed green salad and a tangy dressing. Toast French bread or dinner rolls to go along. Dessert: Amaretto Freeze.

Marilyn Young
Clarksdale

BLACKENED CATFISH

SERVES: 8

1½ cups butter	1 tablespoon thyme (or more)
2 smashed cloves of garlic	1 tablespoon paprika
¼ cup lemon juice	1 tablespoon chopped
1 teaspoon red pepper	parsley
1 teaspoon black pepper	1 tablespoon chopped chives
1 teaspoon salt	8 catfish fillets

Melt butter in a saucepan. Add garlic and let cook a few seconds until flavor is in butter. Remove garlic. Add rest of ingredients. Remove from heat. (Butter should not be browned). Dip fish fillets in the melted butter sauce coating each fillet thoroughly. Heat an iron skillet or griddle until drops of water dance on it. (Hot) An outside gas grill or fish cooker is recommended because a lot of smoke is generated by cooking the fish. Place the fillet, skin side up, on the griddle or skillet for two minutes, turn and cook for an additional two minutes. Remove to serving platter. Cook unused butter sauce until brown, bubbly and slightly thickened. Serve over fillets. Garnish with thinly sliced lemon.

Alex Gates
Sumner

THE ORIGINAL CATFISH NOLAN

YIELD: 4   OVEN: 475°

2 to 2½ pounds catfish fillets	3 to 4 teaspoons fresh garlic
Salt and pepper to taste	in oil
¾ cup bread crumbs	Worcestershire sauce to taste
3 fresh lemons, divided	1 cup crushed pecans
⅓ cup melted butter	

Sprinkle both sides of fish with salt and pepper to taste. Then roll in bread crumbs. Place on greased cookie sheet. Squeeze half a lemon on each fillet; squeeze remaining lemons into melted butter and set aside. Sprinkle fish liberally with garlic then Worcestershire sauce. Bake for 10 minutes or until about one half cooked. Remove from oven and cover with crushed pecans. Return to oven until pecans begin to toast. Do not overcook. Pour lemon butter over fillets and serve.

Nolan Branton and Conley Sullivan
Greenville

CAROLYN'S PAN FRIED CATFISH

SERVES: 4

Teflon skillet (an absolute
   must for this dish)

4 catfish fillets
¼ cup lemon juice

Season the fillets with seasonings of your choice.

SUGGESTED COMBINATIONS:
1. Salt and paprika (my favorite)
2. Salt and lemon pepper
3. Season all
4. Salt, pepper, garlic powder

Heat teflon skillet on medium heat; add fish and pan sauté uncovered for six to eight minutes. Turn over and cook other side six to eight minutes. The fish will be crisp and sometimes blackened depending on the seasoning used. Remove fish from skillet and place on serving plate. Lower heat and add lemon juice. Stir to make sauce then strain over fish. Serve.

Family Secret: Serve fish with baked potato and vegetable.

Carolyn Stringer
Clarksdale

"CATS' MEOW" CATFISH BAKE

SERVES: 8   OVEN: 400°

1½ cups mayonnaise
1 tablespoon creole mustard
1 tablespoon lemon juice
1 tablespoon hot sauce
1 tablespoon Worcestershire
   sauce

2 teaspoons garlic powder
¾ teaspoon curry powder
Buttered crackers
8 fish fillets

Mix first seven ingredients well and spread over eight fish fillets. Sprinkle with crumbled buttered crackers and bake uncovered for about 20 minutes.

Gay Flowers
Mattson

Donna Surholt
Clarksdale

NEW ORLEANS STYLE CATFISH

SERVES: 12 OR 24   OVEN: 350°

1 (8 ounce) can tomato sauce
1 tablespoon vinegar
2 tablespoons salad oil
1 teaspoon garlic powder
1 teaspoon onion salt
1 teaspoon celery salt
½ teaspoon paprika

1 tablespoon Parmesan
cheese
3 tablespoons parsley flakes
1 teaspoon lemon pepper
12 whole catfish or 24 fillets
Salt and pepper

Mix first 10 ingredients and brush on fish. Salt and pepper to taste. Place fish in greased shallow pan. Sprinkle with additional Parmesan cheese. Bake for 40 minutes. Then broil for 3 minutes to brown top.

Georgia Antici
Clarksdale

CATFISH IN SHELLS

SERVES: 8   OVEN: 350°

8 tablespoons margarine
8 tablespoons flour
3 cups milk
4 tablespoons lemon juice
6 tablespoons grated onion
6 tablespoons dried parsley

1⅛ teaspoons salt
¼ teaspoon pepper
Red pepper to taste
Smoked catfish fillets (8
minced)

Melt margarine in saucepan. Stir in flour. Gradually add milk, stirring constantly. Cook until thickened. Add juice, onion, and parsley. Adjust salt, pepper, and red pepper to taste. Add smoked catfish fillets. Put in crab shells and top with buttered bread crumbs and bake 20 minutes or until bubbly. Top with grated cheese and let it melt.

Family Secret: You may substitute crab meat or shrimp for catfish.

Harvey Fiser
Clarksdale

Health Secret: With the exception of shrimp, shellfish are lower in cholesterol and saturated fat per serving than lean beef or skinned chicken. Prepare them boiled or baked without high - fat sauces.

STUFFED CATFISH

SERVES: 6   OVEN: 425°

¾ cup minced celery
½ cup minced onion
½ cup minced fresh parsley
¼ cup minced shallots
¼ cup minced green pepper
1 clove garlic, minced
½ cup butter, melted
1 tablespoon all-purpose
   flour
½ cup milk

½ cup dry white wine
½ pound fresh lump
   crabmeat
1¼ cups seasoned dry bread
   crumbs
¼ teaspoon salt
Dash of pepper
6 (8 ounce) fillets cut in half
   crosswise (catfish of
   course!)

Sauté celery, onion, parsley, shallots, green pepper and garlic in butter in a large skillet over medium heat. Cook until tender. Add flour, cook 2 minutes, stirring constantly. Gradually add milk and wine and cook stirring constantly until thickened. Remove from heat; stir in crab, breadcrumbs, salt and pepper. Place 6 fillets in greased pan; spoon ½ cup crabmeat on each fillet. Cut remaining fillets in half lengthwise. Place fillet fourths on each side of stuffed fillets. Top each with Mornay Sauce. Sprinkle with paprika and bake for 15 to 20 minutes or until fish flakes easily.

MORNAY SAUCE:
YIELD: 2¼ CUPS

¼ cup butter
¼ cup all-purpose flour
2 cups milk
½ teaspoon salt
⅛ teaspoon white pepper

2 egg yolks
1 tablespoon whipping
   cream
¼ cup (1 ounce) shredded
   Swiss cheese

Melt butter in heavy 2 quart saucepan. Add flour stirring until smooth. Cook 1 minute stirring constantly. Gradually add milk and cook over medium heat until thick and bubbly. Stir in salt and pepper. Beat egg yolks until thick and lemon colored. Stir in whipping cream. Gradually stir about ¼ of hot mixture into yolks; add to remaining hot mixture and cook stirring until thickened (2 to 3 minutes). Add cheese and stir until melted. Remove from heat.

Mrs. John Baker
Tutwiler

CARY'S GREAT BAKED FISH

SERVES: 8   OVEN: 375°

2 cups seasoned bread   ¼ teaspoon oregano
  crumbs   ¼ teaspoon basil
¾ cup Parmesan cheese   ½ teaspoon pepper
¼ cup parsley, chopped   ¾ cup margarine, melted
1 teaspoon paprika   8 fish fillets
½ teaspoon salt

Mix all dry ingredients. Dip fish in margarine then in crumbs. Bake
for 25 minutes.

Cary Cocke
Clarksdale

CATFISH IN SHRIMP BOIL

YIELD: 2

2 to 3 catfish fillets

MARINADE:
Juice of 1 lemon   1 teaspoon shrimp boil
Same amount white wine   2 teaspoons lemon pepper
1 teaspoon garlic powder   2 teaspoons dried parsley

Mix marinade and marinate fish all day. Flour fish and pan fry in 2
tablespoons margarine and 2 tablespoons olive oil.

Harvey Fiser and Martha McDonald
Clarksdale

TUNA CROQUETTES

SERVES: 4   OVEN: 450°

1 (6½ ounce) can tuna, flaked 4 tablespoons mayonnaise
½ teaspoon salt   ¼ teaspoon pepper
1 small onion, grated   Cracker crumbs
2 slices bread, crumbled

Mix first six ingredients together and form small croquettes. Roll in
cracker crumbs and bake for 20 minutes.

Georgia Haaga
Clarksdale

SALMON CROQUETTES

My great-great grandmother was making these croquettes in 1903!

SERVES: 6 TO 8

1 medium or 2 small red potatoes	1 egg
1 (15½ ounce) can pink salmon	1½ cups flour
	1 teaspoon salt
1 medium onion, chopped	½ teaspoon black pepper

Boil potatoes with the jackets on until done. In medium bowl remove bones and dark skin from salmon. Remove skin from potatoes and add to salmon, mashing with a fork. Add chopped onion and egg, mixing well. Shape into 8 balls. Mix flour, salt and pepper in pie pan. Roll balls in seasoned flour until well coated. Preheat skillet with ¼ to ½ inch oil. Flatten balls into patties about 1 inch thick. Cook 4 at a time until nicely browned, turning once.

Mrs. T. J. Cassiday, Jr.

BARBECUED SHRIMP A LA BOURBON

YIELD: 6   OVEN: 300°

2 pounds jumbo shrimp	1 (16 ounce) bottle zesty Italian salad dressing
2 cups prepared barbecue sauce	3 tablespoons bourbon whiskey
6 tablespoons freshly squeezed lemon juice	
2 tablespoons Worcestershire sauce	

Chill the shrimp and make your marinade by blending the barbeque sauce, lemon juice, Worcestershire sauce, salad dressing and bourbon over low heat on stove top. It comes out best if you simmer these ingredients for about 10 minutes, uncovered. The alcohol in the bourbon and the vinegar in the salad dressing cook out leaving only the flavoring. Set aside the marinade to cool so that it won't cook your shrimp. Pour the sauce over the shrimp and put in the refrigerator for 4 hours minimum. The longer they marinate the better they will taste. Cook for 40 minutes or until shells start to separate from the tail.

Mrs. Sherry Morris Eason
Mattson

SHRIMP ARTICHOKE CASSEROLE

SERVES: 8   OVEN: 350°

2½ pounds large shrimp   2 (14 ounce) cans artichokes
  (cooked and peeled)   (chopped)

Put peeled shrimp and chopped artichokes in 9 inch x 13 inch greased casserole and pour sauce over. Bake until bubbly or 20 to 30 minutes. Serve over rice, or angel hair pasta.

WHITE SAUCE:
3 tablespoons butter   2 cups sharp cheese, grated
4 tablespoons flour   ½ teaspoon paprika
1 pint half and half cream   1 teaspoon salt
3 tablespoons catsup   ¼ teaspoon red pepper
½ cup sherry   1 tablespoon Worcestershire
1 tablespoon lemon juice   sauce

Make white sauce by melting butter in saucepan. Add flour and blend well. Add half and half cream gradually, stirring constantly. Add other ingredients to white sauce.

Lucy Frye
Clarksdale

Sherry Eason
Matson

Add 2 cans sliced mushroom or fresh mushrooms.

Eva Connell, Virginia Bramlett
Clarksdale

SHRIMP CREOLE CASSEROLE

SERVES: 8   OVEN: 350°

3 pounds shrimp - cooked   ½ cup chopped green pepper
  and peeled, deveined   1 (8 ounce) can mushrooms
1 cup uncooked rice   and juice
½ cup chopped celery   1 (10¾ ounce) can tomato
¼ cup margarine   soup
½ cup chopped onion   1 pound sharp cheese, grated

Sauté onion, green pepper, celery in margarine. Cook rice. Mix all ingredients (save 1 cup cheese for top.) Bake in 2 quart casserole for 45 minutes.

Mrs. Harris Barnes, Jr.
Clarksdale

SHRIMP CANTONESE

SERVES: 4 TO 6

3 or 4 tablespoons oil
½ teaspoon salt
1 whole clove garlic
1 pound medium shrimp,
  shelled and cleaned
½ pound pork, ground or
  chopped fine
1½ cups chicken broth
Dash of pepper

2 teaspoons soy sauce
2 teaspoons cooking sherry
1 tablespoon cornstarch
  mixed with 2 tablespoons
  water
1 egg, slightly beaten
½ teaspoon sesame oil
2 to 3 green onions, chopped

Heat oil in frying pan or wok until hot. Add salt and garlic. Cook for 1 minute being careful not to let garlic burn. Add shrimp. Remove shrimp as soon as it turns pink in color. Remove and discard garlic. Add ground pork to pan and cook until pork is white in color. Add chicken broth, pepper, soy sauce and sherry. Stir and let come to a boil. Return shrimp to pan, stir-fry to mix. Add cornstarch mixture to thicken gravy. Pour beaten egg over shrimp and stir-fry just until egg is set. Stir in sesame oil. Sprinkle cut green onions on top and serve over rice.

Family Secret: Lobster or crab may be used instead of shrimp.

Alice Chow
Clarksdale

BUTTERFLY SHRIMP

SERVES: 3 TO 4

1 cup self-rising flour
½ cup cornstarch
1 teaspoon salt
1 teaspoon black pepper
½ teaspoon monosodium
  glutamate

1 egg
12 (26/30) sized shrimp
12 (3 inch) strips of bacon

Combine flour, cornstarch, salt, pepper, and monosodium glutamate into a 9 inch x 13 inch pan. Mix thoroughly. In a small bowl, beat egg for 15 to 20 seconds or until egg is smooth. Slice shrimp along the back, but not completely through. Remove the black vein that follows along the back and rinse shrimp in water. Dip shrimp in the egg. Place 1 shrimp on 1 strip of bacon. Dredge in flour mixture, holding shrimp-bacon together. Fry in deep fryer for 3 minutes. Serve immediately.

Jean Wong
Clarksdale

SZECHUAN JADEITE PRAWNS

SERVES: 2 TO 3

8 to 12 ounces peeled fresh
  prawns or shrimp
2 egg whites, lightly beaten
1 tablespoon cornstarch
Pinch of salt
3 to 5 tablespoons oil for
  frying

½ cup frozen green peas
1 green onion
1 pickled red chili, finely
  chopped

Devein the prawns. Rinse in cold water after rubbing with a little cornstarch and salt to whiten. Dry on paper towels and place in a dish, adding the egg whites, cornstarch, and pinch of salt. Mix well and let stand for 20 minutes. Heat the oil in a wok and stir-fry the prawns a few minutes over high heat until cooked through, then remove from wok. Add the peas, green onion and chili to the wok and stir-fry for one minute; then add the sauce ingredients, except the cornstarch and a little of the stock. Cover and simmer until peas are tender (few minutes). Return the prawns. Mix cornstarch with the remaining stock, pour into the sauce and simmer, stirring, until thickened and clear. Serve at once.

SAUCE:
1 cup chicken broth
1 teaspoon rice wine or dry
  sherry

¾ teaspoon salt
Pinch of white pepper
1 tablespoon cornstarch

Mamie Pang
Marks

SHRIMP MORNAY OVER ANGEL HAIR PASTA

SERVES: 6

5 tablespoons butter
4 tablespoons all-purpose
  flour
4 tablespoons green onion,
  chopped
1 (4 ounce) can mushrooms
1 pint half and half
1 tablespoon Worcestershire
  sauce
1 tablespoon lemon juice
½ cup white wine

2 egg yolks
½ cup grated Swiss cheese
¼ cup Parmesan cheese
¼ teaspoon red pepper
½ teaspoon salt
White pepper to taste
1 pound shrimp, boiled and
  peeled
1 (9 ounce) package fresh
  Angel Hair Pasta

CONTINUED, SHRIMP MORNAY OVER ANGEL HAIR PASTA

Melt butter and sauté green onions and mushrooms. Add flour, stirring until smooth. Cook 1 minute stirring constantly. Gradually add half and half, wine, Worcestershire sauce and lemon juice and cook over medium heat until thick and bubbly. Beat egg yolks and add to sauce; be sure to add a little of hot mixture to egg yolks before adding eggs to the sauce. Add cheeses, salt and pepper and shrimp and simmer for 5 minutes. Cook pasta according to the package directions. Drain and put on a platter. Pour sauce over pasta and serve. I usually find the fresh angel hair pasta in the deli area of Krogers.

Sherry M. Eason
Mattson

BEIJING TOMATO PRAWN CAKES

SERVES: 4

PRAWN CAKES:

1 pound fresh shrimp	1 teaspoon finely chopped
2 egg whites	ginger (optional)
1 tablespoon cornstarch	Oil for deep frying

Peel and devein the prawns. Rinse in cold water, drain and pat dry with a paper towel. Grind in a food processor. Beat egg whites until frothy and add the cornstarch and ginger. Mix with the prawns and stir the mixture in one direction only until thoroughly mixed and smooth. Heat the oil in a wok or deep fryer; form spoonfuls of the prawn mixture into coin-shaped pieces, and deep-fry over moderate heat until golden. Remove. Place in a strainer and drain well.

SWEET AND SOUR SAUCE:

½ cup chicken broth	2 tablespoons rice wine or
½ cup sugar	dry sherry
4 tablespoons vinegar	1 tablespoon cornstarch
3 tablespoons tomato catsup	¾ teaspoon salt

In a saucepan, mix the sauce ingredients and bring to a boil, stirring constantly, until thickened; then simmer for another minute. Arrange the prawn cakes on a plate and pour the sauce over them before serving.

Seng Pang
Clarksdale

SHRIMP, BUFFET STYLE

SERVES: 10 TO 12

5 pounds shrimp
3 cups mayonnaise
Juice of 3 lemons
6 thin slices of onion, rings
    separated
Cracked seasoned pepper

Seasoned salt
Hot sauce
Red pepper
⅓ cup chopped fresh parsley
2 cans pineapple chunks,
    (optional)

Cook raw shrimp until just tender. Combine mayonnaise and lemon juice and condiments. Use generous amounts of seasoning. Mix mayonnaise mixture with shrimp, onions, and parsley. Marinate for 24 hours. If desired, fold in pineapple chunks when served. This adds a fresh taste. Sprinkle extra chopped parsley on top to add color. This shrimp can be served with crackers and/or toothpicks at a buffet affair. Also, could be used to stuff tomatoes or avocadoes for a salad.

Family Secret: Whenever I have served this shrimp to a large gathering, it was always completely consumed. I added the pineapple to stretch the recipe and found it was an interesting and enjoyable addition.

Tonya T. Marley
Sumner

SEAFOOD GUMBO

SERVES: 12

1 cup bacon grease or
    vegetable oil
1 cup all-purpose flour
2 onions, chopped
2 bell peppers, chopped
2 cloves garlic, chopped
1 stalk celery, chopped
8 cups water
2 (8 ounce) cans tomato sauce

1 tablespoon soy sauce
3 bay leaves
3 teaspoons thyme
Salt and pepper to taste
1 bag crab boil
1 pound crab meat
2 pounds shrimp
Oysters, optional

Heat bacon grease and flour to make roux. Stir constantly until flour is VERY brown. Add chopped vegetables and cook in roux until limp. Then add water, tomato sauce, and seasonings. Put in the bag of crab boil. Simmer 3 to 4 hours. Add seafood 30 minutes before serving. Serve on rice and sprinkle with gumbo filé.

Mrs. Rick Parsons
Sumner

SHRIMP AND WILD RICE

SERVES: 12   OVEN: 300°

½ cup all-purpose flour
1 cup margarine, melted
   (divided)
4 cups chicken broth
¼ teaspoon pepper
1 cup chopped onion
½ cup chopped green pepper
1 (6 ounce) can sliced
   mushrooms

3½ pounds shrimp, cooked,
   peeled and deveined
2 tablespoons Worcestershire
   sauce
Hot sauce to taste
5 cups cooked long grain
   wild rice

Gradually add flour to ½ cup melted margarine. Cook over low heat, stirring constantly, until it bubbles. Add broth gradually and cook until smooth and thickened, continuing to stir. Add pepper and simmer two to three minutes more. Sauté onion, green pepper and mushrooms in remaining margarine. Drain and combine with white sauce and remaining ingredients. Spoon into 2-quart casserole and bake for 45-50 minutes.

Jeannine White
Clarksdale

SHRIMP STROGANOFF

SERVES: 6 TO 8

1½ to 2 pounds shelled and
   deveined medium shrimp
6 tablespoons melted margarine
1½ cups sliced mushrooms
2 tablespoons minced onion
1 clove minced garlic

3 tablespoons flour
1 to 2 cups chicken broth
1 teaspoon catsup
1 cup sour cream
½ teaspoon Worcestershire
   sauce

Cook shrimp in 3 tablespoons (or more) margarine for 3-5 minutes, turning often. Remove and keep warm. Add mushrooms to 3 tablespoons margarine and sauté for 2 minutes. Add onion and garlic and sauté until tender. Add more margarine if needed. Stir in flour and broth and cook until thickened. Add catsup and Worcestershire. Remove from heat and add sour cream and shrimp. Serve over rice!

Barbara B. Graves
Clarksdale

SPINACH AND OYSTER CASSEROLE

YIELD: 4 TO 6   OVEN: 350°

2 (10 ounce) boxes chopped
   frozen spinach
4 tablespoons butter or
   margarine
2 tablespoons flour
2 tablespoons onions,
   chopped
½ cup evaporated milk
½ cup liquor of cooked
   spinach

½ teaspoon black pepper
¾ teaspoon celery salt
½ teaspoon salt
1 roll jalapeño cheese
1 teaspoon Worcestershire
   sauce
1 pint oysters
½ cup cracker crumbs
   (optional)

Cook spinach by directions, reserving liquor. Set aside to drain.
Melt butter and stir in flour. Add onions and cook until soft. Add
milk, liquor, and seasonings; cook to a sauce consistency. Cook
oysters in own juice until they curl. Cut up and pour off juice. Add
spinach and oysters to sauce mixture. Blend and put in 1½ quart
casserole. May top with cracker crumbs, if desired, and bake until
bubbly in center.

Family Secret: This dish is an elegant addition for a cocktail buffet.
It is fully cooked, so the baking can be eliminated. Serve in a silver
chafing dish with melba toast or toasted bread quarters.

Marty Laney
Lyon

Health Secret: Dry your fresh herbs in the microwave. Try
including oregano, rosemary, sage, savory, tarragon, thyme and
mint. Parsley and basil do NOT hold their flavor well. Wash and
dry freshly picked herbs. Arrange in single layer on paper towels.
Microwave on high until leaves shrivel, about 1 to 3 minutes. Let
stand overnight and then store in air tight container.

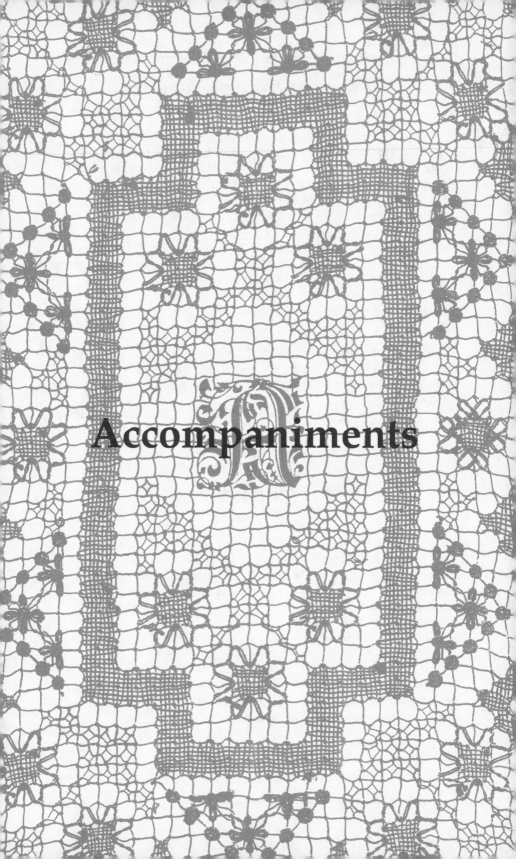

Accompaniments

FETTUCINI ALL' ALFREDO

SERVES: 4 TO 6   OVEN: 350°

1 pound egg noodles -
   medium width
½ cup butter
¼ to ½ cup warm cream or
   half and half

1½ to 2 cups fresh, finely
   grated Parmesan cheese
Freshly ground black pepper
   (coarsely ground)

Set large pot salted water to boil. Set oven at 350°. Place butter in oven proof dish, allow to melt - NOT BROWN. Boil noodles 8 to 9 minutes; DRAIN. Remove hot dish from oven. Add pasta. Toss with 2 spoons. Add cream and toss. Move pasta to one side, liquid should be seeping around edges. Add cheese, gradually tossing as you add. Add pepper. Serve immediately.

Family Secret: Pass up the grated cheese on the grocer's shelf and buy a block of Parmesan cheese and grate it at home. You will really be surprised at the difference!! Cut it in chunks and put in food processor.

Charley Connerly
Clarksdale

TONI'S TORTELLINI

SERVES: 4

1 (7 ounce) box tortellini
1 (4 ounce) wedge Parmesan
   grated
½ pint half and half
¼ cup butter
1 can artichoke hearts,
   quartered

10 to 12 fresh mushrooms,
   chopped and sautéed
2 zucchini, sliced and
   sautéed

In salted boiling water (2 tablespoons of salt) cook tortellini by package directions. Drain. Add butter. Add cheese; toss until melted. Add cream, artichokes, mushrooms, and zucchini.

Toni Hardin
Duncan

NOODLE CASSEROLE

In the early days of Jewish history, Noodle Casserole or "Lukchen Kugel" was prepared on the festival of Shabuot, the traditional birthday of the Torah, or Law. On this holiday dairy foods are traditionally eaten because the Torah is compared to "milk and honey".

YIELD: 15   OVEN: 400°

½ cup margarine
16 ounce wide egg noodles,
   cooked and drained
1 cup sour cream
3 cups cottage cheese
4 tablespoons sugar

4 eggs
½ cup sugar
1½ cups milk
1 teaspoon vanilla flavoring
1 cup raisins (optional)
Cinnamon-sugar

Melt margarine in oblong 3 quart casserole. Cook noodles in rapidly boiling salted water for about 10 minutes; drain. Add to melted margarine in pyrex dish. Combine next three ingredients and mix them well into the noodles. Beat eggs, sugar, mild and vanilla together and pour this over the sugar noodles. Refrigerate overnight. Before baking, mix in raisins and sprinkle top generously with cinnamon-sugar. Bake uncovered in preheated oven until brown on top or about 1 hour. Cut into squares and serve hot. Can be baked and frozen.

Family Secret: This casserole is very versatile. It may be served with fresh fruit and bagels for breakfast, with chicken salad and marinated vegetables for lunch, or with broiled chicken and salad for dinner.

Goldie Hirsberg
Clarksdale

RISSOTO ALLA VILANESE

SERVES: 8 TO 10

⅛ pound salt pork, chopped fine
⅛ pound beef fat, chopped fine
¼ cup butter
1 medium gizzard, chopped fine
4 chicken livers, chopped fine
1 package dried mushrooms boiled in ½ cup water, drained and chopped fine
1½ pounds rice
3 (12 ounce) cans chicken broth
1 capsule saffron (soaked in ½ cup hot chicken broth)
Parmesan cheese

Brown salt pork and beef in butter. Add onions and add mushrooms. Sauté 5 minutes. Add liver, gizzards; sauté 10 minutes. Add rice, salt and pepper to taste. Boil broth and ladle in a little at at time, stirring frequently. (May not need all of broth. Should not be soupy.) Rice will be done in about 18 minutes. When rice is half done, add saffron and broth it's soaking in. Sprinkle generously with Parmesan cheese.

Toni Malvezzi Hardin
Duncan

SADIE ROSSIE'S LEBANESE RICE

½ cup broken thin spaghetti
½ cup butter or margarine
2 cups uncooked long grain rice
2 cups chicken broth
2 cups hot water
¼ teaspoon ground cinnamon
1 teaspoon each salt and pepper

Fry spaghetti in butter until brown. Add rice and sauté for two minutes. Add chicken broth, water, cinnamon, salt and pepper. Cook on high for 5 minutes. After it starts to boil, cover and cook on low heat for about 20 minutes. Do not stir; it will cook down. Serve with baked chicken and a Lebanese salad.

Yvonne Rossie Abraham
Clarksdale

RICE SUPREME

SERVES: 6   OVEN: 375°

2 (10½ ounce) cans beef   1 cup raw rice
  bouillon   1 (4 ounce) can mushrooms
½ cup butter, melted

Mix all ingredients in a 2 quart casserole. Season well with salt and pepper. Bake one hour covered. Uncover and bake 15 more minutes or until top is brown and rice is cooked. You may use consommé instead of bouillon.

Family Secret: This rice dish is so easy to make and is wonderful for company because you can stick it in the oven and don't have to worry about rice sticking or flopping! Great with wild game or steak!

Gay Flowers
Dublin

Variation: Use 1 can beef bouillon and 1 can French onion soup.

Sherry Eason
Mattson

LENTILS WITH RICE (IMJADARA' ROZ)

SERVES: 6 TO 10

1 cup lentils   1 cup long grain rice
Water   1 large onion
1 teaspoon salt   ½ cup oil
½ teaspoon black pepper

Check lentils for any foreign matter. Wash thoroughly. Put in a 2 quart boiler. Bring to boil. Drain and rinse. Return to boiler with 1 quart of water. Bring to boil again. Add salt, pepper, and rice. While rice and beans are cooking, brown chopped or thinly sliced onions in oil in skillet. Add oil to rice mixture and use onions to garnish top when served, or stir both onions and oil into rice mixture.

Yvonne Rossie Abraham
Clarksdale

FRIED RICE

SERVES: 4 TO 6

2 tablespoons vegetable oil
1 cup diced barbecued pork (roast pork) may be purchased at Chinese deli or restaurant - ham may be substituted
¼ cup diced green onion
4 cups cold cooked long grain rice

½ cup frozen peas (cooked)
½ cup diced celery
Pepper to taste
½ teaspoon salt
1½ tablespoons soy sauce
2 eggs, beaten
Several drops of sesame oil (no substitute - may be bought in Chinese grocery)

In a preheated wok or skillet, place 2 tablespoons oil. Turn to high heat, stir-fry pork and onion for 1 minute, then add rice along with peas, celery, pepper, salt, and soy sauce. Press rice gently into pan with a large spatula and fry for a few seconds, repeating the process until the rice is hot clear through. Turn and mix rapidly for 5 minutes. Add a few drops of vegetable oil if necessary to prevent burning. Add eggs. Mix and toss until eggs are done, about 1 minute. Add sesame oil. Just before serving, toss.

Gilroy Chow
Clarksdale

EVELYN'S CORNBREAD DRESSING

Evelyn has cooked for my brother's family for 35 years. The whole family has used this recipe and none other!

SERVES: 8   OVEN: 350°

4 cups cornbread pieces
4 cups toasted bread pieces
2 cups chicken stock
4 eggs
1 cup chopped celery
1 cup chopped onions

½ pound hot sausage, crumbled, browned, and drained
2 teaspoons salt
2 teaspoons pepper

Mix cornbread and bread with broth, then add other ingredients and mix with hands until completely mixed. Pour into a greased 8 x 8 inch pan and bake for thirty minutes, uncovered. When done, cut into squares. (This is not a soft dressing.) It's hot but great!

Family Secret: It can be easily doubled and freezes well.

Mrs. Graham Bramlett
Clarksdale

RIPIENO ("P" OR GREEN STUFFING)

"P" is short for "Ripieno" which means "stuffed". It is, of course, the green stuffing served with turkey.

YIELD: ABOUT 6 OR 7 CUPS   OVEN: 350°

1 cup chopped celery
1 cup chopped carrots
1 cup chopped onion
2 cloves garlic, minced
1 tablespoon each butter and
   olive oil
1 (10 ounce) package frozen
   chopped spinach

6 each chicken livers and
   gizzards
2½ cups grated Parmesan
   cheese
2 cups bread crumbs
8 to 9 eggs, slightly beaten
Salt and pepper to taste

Sauté celery, onion, garlic and carrots in butter and olive oil. Prepare spinach according to package directions. Boil chicken liver and gizzards about 15 minutes and chip fine. In a large bowl combine sautéed vegetables, spinach, and chopped livers and gizzards. Add Parmesan cheese, bread crumbs, eggs, and salt and pepper. Mix well. Use as stuffing for turkey, chicken, artichokes or wild game.

Family Secret: This recipe can be doubled or tripled and frozen for later use. It does swell during cooking. If not used as stuffing it can be baked separately in an oblong pan at 350° for 1 hour.

Celeste C. Wise
Clarksdale

SPOON BREAD

SERVES: 4   OVEN: 400°

1 cup salted cooked grits
¼ cup margarine

1 cup milk
2 beaten eggs

Mix first 3 ingredients while grits are hot. Add egg when slightly cooled. Pour into a casserole dish and cook until brown or approximately 30 minutes.

Sherry Donald
Clarksdale

POLENTA (PLANTA)

Carol's grandmother, Mrs. A. Noe, always made this in the winter since it warms your whole body.

SERVES: 4 TO 6

7 cups water
2 teaspoons salt

3 cups plain meal

Let water (with salt) come to a boil, then turn heat down to simmer. Gradually add meal while continously stirring. Must use wooden spoon. When all meal has been added turn heat to medium. Continue to stir and fold meal mixture until mixture pulls from side of pan. This usually takes about 10 minutes. Immediately turn onto cutting board and mold into a mound using a moist soup bowl. Let cool completely. Slice ¼ inch thick (any length desired) and place in a cool skillet with small amount of shortening. Using medium heat fry until crispy brown on one side. Turn and fry other side the same. Drain and immediately serve topped with spaghetti sauce and grated Cheddar cheese. May be served plain or with slice of Cheddar cheese between two slices of Planta. Wrap portion that hasn't been fried in clean dish cloth or plastic wrap and keep refrigerated.

Carol Andrews
Clarksdale

Variation: After frying until golden brown, spoon Stufado (Wild Ducks in Wine) over Polenta and serve.

Toni Carol Hardin
Duncan

CUSH

No one seems to know the origin of the name "cush", but the dish originated as a use for left-over cornbread and biscuits.

SERVES: 5 TO 6   OVEN: 350°

2 tablespoons drippings
2 tablespoons butter
3 cups cornbread and
   biscuits (more cornbread
   than biscuits)
Salt and pepper

1 teaspoon sage or poultry
   seasoning
1 chopped onion
2 eggs
Sweet milk

Heat drippings and butter in heavy skillet. Break up cold cornbread and biscuits. Add to hot fat with onions, salt, pepper, sage and beaten eggs. Stir and brown lightly. Then add milk to make a soft mushy batter and cook until fairly dry - or may be baked in 1 quart dish (I prefer this) for 20 to 30 minutes.

Margaret S. Craig
Friars Point

CHEESE APPLES

SERVES: 6 TO 8   OVEN: 350°

¾ cup sugar
½ cup flour
¼ teaspoon salt
¼ cup butter
1 cup sharp shredded
   Cheddar cheese

7 medium size tart apples,
   peeled and sliced
6 tablespoons water
1 tablespoon lemon juice

Combine sugar, flour, and salt. Cut butter into mixture until coarse crumbs form. Add 1 cup sharp shredded cheese. Set aside. Combine sliced apples (peeling is optional), water, and lemon juice. Toss to coat apples and keep them from turning brown. Spoon into 8 inch square dish. Sprinkle cheese mixture over and pat down gently. Bake for forty minutes.

Family Secret: Granny Smith apples make this dish especially good. It is wonderful served with pork.

Mrs. Hartley Kittle (Lynn)
Clarksdale

CRANBERRY APPLE CASSEROLE

SERVES: 8   OVEN: 325°

3 cups peeled and chopped
   apples
2 cups fresh cranberries
¾ cup sugar

⅓ cup dark brown sugar
½ cup margarine, melted
¾ cup oatmeal
⅓ cup pecans, chopped

Mix apples, cranberries, and sugar and spread in a 1½ quart oblong dish. Mix together the brown sugar, margarine, oatmeal, and pecans, and spread on top. Bake for 45 minutes.

Family Secret: This is a tasty, colorful fruit dish that is especially good with turkey and dressing.

Mrs. Rick Parsons
Sumner

EASY HOT FRUIT

SERVES: 8 TO 10   OVEN: 300°

⅓ cup butter
¾ cup brown sugar
1 (16 ounce) can applesauce
1 (16 ounce) can pineapple
  chunks, drained
1 (8 ounce) jar cherries, cut in
  half

4 bananas, sliced
1 (1 pound 13 ounce) can
  peaches, cut up and
  drained
1 cup chopped pecans

Melt butter and add brown sugar and applesauce. Add all fruit and pour in 2½ quart casserole. Top with pecans. Bake about 30 minutes until bubbly.

Family Secret: This is wonderful with almost any meat but really "hits the spot" with ham.

Mrs. Bill Luckett, Jr. (Francine)
Clarksdale

BAKED PINEAPPLE AND CHEESE

SERVES: 6 TO 8   OVEN: 350°

1 (20 ounce) can chunk
  pineapple
1 cup shredded sharp
  Cheddar cheese
3 tablespoons flour
3 tablespoons pineapple
  juice

½ cup sugar
¾ cup crumbled butter
  crackers
¼ cup margarine, melted

Drain pineapple and reserve juice. Place pineapple in mixing bowl and add shredded Cheddar cheese. Mix flour, sugar, and juice. Add to pineapple and stir well. Place in an 8 inch square pyrex dish that has been oiled. Mix crackers and margarine and sprinkle over pineapple. Bake 30 minutes.

Family Secret: Very good with ham, turkey, or game.

Nan M. Russell
Jonestown

ASPARAGUS CASSEROLE

SERVES: 4 TO 6   OVEN: 350°

2 tablespoons margarine
2 tablespoons asparagus
  juice
1 scant cup milk
½ teaspoon pepper
½ teaspoon salt
1 teaspoon paprika
Red pepper to taste

¾ pound sharp Cheddar
  cheese, grated
1 (6 ounce) can sliced
  mushrooms
2 (15 ounce) cans asparagus
  spears
2 hard-cooked eggs, sliced
Slivered almonds

Drain asparagus, save juice. Melt margarine, add flour, mix well. Add asparagus juice, making a paste. Return to heat; add milk, stirring constantly. Season with salt, pepper, paprika and red pepper. Add cheese; stir until dissolved. Add mushrooms. Line bottom of 3 quart casserole with 1 can asparagus. Cover with half of cheese sauce and 1 egg. Repeat and top with almonds. Bake for 20 minutes.

Pat Mitchell
Clarksdale

FRESH GREEN BEANS

SERVES: 8

2 pounds fresh green beans
1 medium onion, chopped
2 cloves garlic, minced

Salt and pepper to taste
Non-sticking spray

Clean and snap beans. Spray pot with the non-sticking spray, generously. Sauté green beans, onions and garlic about 10 to 15 minutes. Add hot water to cover beans and cook covered on lowest temperature until beans are cooked to the desired doneness. Use this same technique for butter beans and purple hull peas. This has no added fat.

Carolyn Stringer
Clarksdale

Health Secret: Losses of vitamin C are less in fruits and vegetables cooked by microwave instead of by conventional methods.

GREEN BEAN CASSEROLE

SERVES: 6   OVEN: 350°

2 (10 ounce) packages frozen,   ¼ cup melted butter or
  French-cut green beans   margarine
1 cup sliced, fresh   ½ cup grated Parmesan
  mushrooms   cheese
1 cup sliced water chestnuts   4 round butter crackers,
½ cup chopped pimento   crushed fine
1 teaspoon soy sauce
1 can cream of mushroom
  soup, undiluted

Cook green beans and drain well. Mix with mushrooms, water chestnuts, pimento, soy sauce, soup, and melted butter. Put into a 2 quart casserole. Sprinkle with Parmesan cheese and crushed crackers. Bake 25 to 30 minutes or until bubbly and brown on top.

Family Secret: I have made this casserole a lot for holiday suppers.

Mrs. Inger H. Flautt
Sumner

HARVARD BEETS

SERVES: 4

⅓ cup sugar   ¼ to ½ teaspoon salt
2 tablespoons flour   2 cups canned beets, sliced
¼ cup water or beet juice   or diced
2 tablespoons margarine

Mix sugar and flour together in saucepan. Add next 5 ingredients. Stir. Cook over medium heat, stirring often till thickened. Add beets and heat thoroughly.

Emily Cooper
Clarksdale

Health Secret: One medium - size red bell pepper contains more than twice the vitamin C of an orange.

ARTICHOKE AND GREEN BEAN CASSEROLE

SERVES: 6   OVEN: 350°

1 can (13¾ ounce) artichokes, drained
⅓ cup liquid from artichokes
1 can (16 ounce) French-cut green beans
¾ cup Italian style bread crumbs

⅓ cup grated Romano cheese
1 tablespoon minced parsley
2 small cloves garlic, minced
4 tablespoons olive oil
Salt and pepper to taste

Chop artichokes; add all ingredients. Mix well. Pour in olive oil-greased glass dish. Cover and bake 30 minutes. Microwave: May be covered with plastic wrap and cooked on medium power for 15 minutes.

Celia Cuicchi
Shaw

ARTICHOKE BOTTOMS
STUFFED WITH SPINACH

SERVES: 10 TO 12   OVEN: 350°

2 cans artichoke bottoms
4 (10 ounce) packages chopped spinach, cooked and drained, squeeze the excess water out
½ cup butter or margarine
1 cup chopped onion

2 tablespoons Worcestershire sauce
2 (10¾) ounce cans cream of mushroom soup
Salt, pepper, and garlic powder to taste
Parmesan cheese

Melt butter and cook onion until clear. Add Worcestershire sauce, soups, and seasonings. Combine with spinach. Fill each artichoke with spinach mixture and place in a single layer in a flat casserole. Sprinkle with cheese and bake until hot, about 15 minutes.

Mrs. Bill Luckett, Jr.
Clarksdale

BAKED BEANS FOR 60

SERVES: 60   OVEN: 300°

4 (52 ounce) cans pork and   3 to 4 bunches of green
  beans   onions, chopped
2 pounds bacon, chopped   ½ (5 ounce) jar mustard
1 (32 ounce bottle) catsup   2 boxes dark brown sugar

Mix all ingredients together and bake 3 to 4 hours. Let sit for 1 hour before serving.

Donna Merkel
Clarksdale

BAKED BEANS MEDLEY

Linda Langston's husband entered this recipe in the Memphis in May barbecue competition in 1987.

YIELD: 10 TO 12   OVEN: 375°

1 pound bacon, cooked and   1 pound (12 ounce can) pork
  crumbled   and beans
3 tablespoons bacon drip-   1 (16 ounce can) lima beans,
  pings (more or less to taste)   drained
1 onion, chopped   1 (16 ounce can) red kidney
1 bell pepper, chopped   beans, drained
1 cup brown sugar   1 (16 ounce can) butter beans,
¼ cup white vinegar   drained
¼ cup water

Cook bacon, drain, and crumble. Sauté onion in 3 tablespoons of drippings. Add sugar, water, and vinegar and simmer until thick. Add all beans and crumbled bacon. Place in 2 quart casserole dish and bake 1 hour.

Family Secret: I like to add ¼ cup of my favorite barbeque sauce. This can also be cooked in a crock pot and will freeze, if needed.

Linda Dulaney
Clarksdale

Health Secret: For picky eaters - whatever their age - try disguising vegetables in foods they like. Shredded carrots or finely chopped broccoli may go completely unnoticed in spaghetti sauce or meatloaf.

NEW YEAR'S DAY BLACKEYE PEAS

I have been handed down an 1845 silver dollar which has only been used for this New Year's Day recipe. For the fun of it, I add 2 new silver dollars to the pot. Whoever gets a new one keeps it and should expect prosperity in the new year.

SERVES: 30

5 (1 pound) packages dry
  blackeye peas
2 pound smoked hog jowl
  (have butcher cut in cubes)

5 peeled garlic cloves; crush,
  do not chop
1 "silver" dollar
2 tablespoons pepper

Soak all the dry peas in the biggest container you have, overnight. For 5 packages of peas I use a gallon of water. The next day drain off any excess water. In a stock pot, (mine is 4 gallons) add 1 gallon water and cut up hog jowl; bring to boil. Add peas - you will need to add more water as it cooks. The peas should be very soupy until last hour of cooking. In the last hour, add your crushed garlic and cover and simmer until peas are tender. The silver is added when you add garlic. Simmer approximately 2 hours.

Family Secret: If hog jowl isn't available, you can use hamhocks or better yet, the leftover bone and meat from a Honey Baked ham. Serve with Bloody Marys, assorted dips and appetizers, slaw, pickled onions, Mexican cornbread, cracklin' cornbread and lemon ice box pie.

Roselyn B. Dulaney
Clarksdale

MARINATED BLACK EYE PEAS

SERVES: 4

2 (20 ounce) cans blackeyed
  peas
1 cup salad oil
¼ cup wine vinegar

1 clove crushed garlic
¼ cup sliced onion
½ teaspoon salt
½ teaspoon pepper

Mix oil, vinegar, and seasonings. Add peas. Marinate overnight. Serve cold.

Linda Hood
Duncan

BROCCOLI AMANDINE CASSEROLE

SERVES: 6 TO 8   OVEN: 350°

1 bunch fresh broccoli or 2
  (10 ounce) packages frozen
  broccoli florets
1 beef bouillon cube
¼ cup hot water
4 tablespoons butter or
  margarine
4 tablespoons flour
2 tablespoons dry sherry

1 cup light cream
2 tablespoons lemon juice
½ teaspoon salt
¼ teaspoon white pepper
½ cup grated Parmesan
  cheese
½ cup grated Gouda cheese
¼ cup sliced almonds, toasted

Cook broccoli in rapidly boiling water until just tender, about 6 minutes. Drain and place in a buttered 2 quart casserole. Dissolve bouillon cube in water. In a 1 quart saucepan, melt butter. Add flour and cook stirring constantly 1 to 2 minutes. Pour in cream and bouillon, beating vigorously with a wire whisk. Bring sauce to a boil and stir until thick and smooth, about 3 to 5 minutes. Remove from heat and add sherry, lemon juice, salt and pepper. Pour sauce over broccoli. Sprinkle with cheese and almonds. Bake 20 minutes.

Sherry Eason
Mattson

EGGPLANT PATTIES

SERVES: 4

2 cups cooked, drained
  eggplant
½ cup minced onion (can use
  green onions)
2 beaten eggs
¼ teaspoon black or white
  pepper

Dash of garlic powder
1 cup crushed cracker
  crumbs
¾ cup corn meal to coat
  patties

Cook and drain eggplant; add onion, eggs, and seasoning. Stir in cracker crumbs. Make into flat patties and lightly pat corn meal on each side before putting patties into hot oil. Fry in ¼ inch of oil and turn only one time. Drain on paper towels. Serve hot.

Roselyn Dulaney
Clarksdale

GRANDMOTHER FREEMAN'S SWEET POTATO CASSEROLE

SERVES: 8 TO 10   OVEN: 350°

8 sweet potatoes (or about 8   ⅓ cup orange juice
   to 10 cups of mashed sweet   1 teaspoon vanilla extract
   potatoes)   1 teaspoon cinnamon
¾ cup margarine   ½ teaspoon nutmeg
2 eggs   Marshmallows, raisins, and
2 cups sugar   chopped nuts (optional)

Peel sweet potatoes and cut up in small pieces and boil until tender. Drain. Then add drained potatoes to a large mixing bowl and add butter to melt in hot potatoes. Whip. Add all rest of ingredients and mix with blender until smooth. (You can add raisins and chopped nuts if you desire). Pour in casserole dish (and top with marshmallows - optional) and cook for about 25 minutes.

Family Secret: The sweet potato mixture can be put in orange halves, topped with a marshmallow and browned under the broiler. A hollowed pumpkin with fluted edge is also a colorful serving bowl.

Meg Agostinelli
Lyon

BOOGA BOTTOM'S EGGPLANT CASSEROLE

SERVES: 8   OVEN: 350°

4 cups raw eggplant or 1   2 eggs (beaten)
   large eggplant   ¼ cup milk
2 chopped onions   ¼ pound cheese
½ teaspoon salt   1 (12½ ounce) can tomatoes
1 teaspoon pepper   1½ cups cracker crumbs
2 tablespoons sugar   ⅓ stick margarine

Peel eggplant, wash, and cut into rounds. Then dice in 1 inch squares. Put in saucepan with chopped onions, salt, pepper, sugar, add just enough water so eggplant is covered (approximately 1½ to 2 cups). Bring to boil, and let sit 5 minutes, drain off liquid. Add egg, milk, cheese, tomatoes to eggplant mixture. Pour mixture into 9 x 13 inch pan. Top with cracker crumbs, then dot with margarine. Bake for 45 minutes, uncovered.

Booga Bottom Store
Duncan

GRILLED STUFFED EGGPLANT

SERVES: 4

2 eggplants
1 fresh tomato
¼ cup chopped fresh parsley
   or 1 teaspoon dried parsley
   flakes

1 clove garlic, minced
½ cup bread crumbs
Salt and pepper
¼ cup oil

Wash and slice eggplants in half lengthwise. Hollow out centers and dice into very small pieces. Peel, chop and dice tomato. Wash parsley and chop finely. Put all ingredients in a large bowl. Add bread crumbs, salt and pepper. Pour oil over all and mix well. Fill eggplant shells with the mixture and cook on charcoal grill with top closed until pulp is soft and bubbly. (About 45 minutes). Shells will flake on bottom but this does not matter since you only eat filling.

Edith Borgognoni
Clarksdale

MUSHROOM CASSEROLE

SERVES: 8 TO 10   OVEN: 350°

½ to ¾ cup margarine or
   more as needed
2 cups fresh sliced
   mushrooms

3 cups cubed fresh tomatoes
4 cups fresh onion, (rings)
1 cup bread crumbs
Dash of garlic salt

Sauté each vegetable separately in margarine; First, mushrooms and set aside; Second, onion rings and set aside; Third, tomatoes and ½ cup bread crumbs and set aside. Layering casserole as: onion rings, tomatoes and crumbs, mushrooms. Sprinkle ¼ cup remaining bread crumbs on this and a little garlic salt. Repeat 3 times and top with remaining crumbs and garlic salt. Cook for 30 to 35 minutes until bubbly.

Lucille Steen
Clarksdale

Health Secret: Do not add baking soda when cooking vegetables; it destroys vitamin C and some B vitamins.

BRAISED CABBAGE

SERVES: 4

1½ pounds shredded cabbage   4 stalks chives
3 grated carrots   Salt and pepper
3 tablespoons butter

In skillet heat butter until foamy. Add chives and sauté until tender. Add green cabbage and carrots. Sauté over high heat until tender but crisp, about 4 minutes. Add salt and pepper to taste. If you don't have any scallions, onions are the next best substitute.

Sue Bell
Clarksdale

FRESH CORN PUDDING

SERVES: 6 TO 8   OVEN: 325°

2 cups fresh young corn (cut   ¼ cup sugar
   off the cob)   ½ teaspoon salt
3 tablespoons butter, melted   ¾ cup half and half
2 eggs, beaten   ¾ cup milk

Mix all together very well. Add corn and any juices from cut corn. Bake for 45 minutes or until pudding is firm. If canned corn is used, add 2 teaspoons flour with the sugar.

Mrs. Lytle McKee (Claudine)
Clarksdale

QUICK CORN SOUFFLÉ

SERVES: 4 TO 6   OVEN: 350°

1 (16½ ounce) can cream   2 tablespoons flour
   style corn   2 eggs, beaten
2 tablespoons sugar   ¼ cup milk

Mix all ingredients and pour into 1 quart pyrex dish which has been greased with margarine. Dot top with margarine pieces. Bake, uncovered, for 30-45 minutes until knife inserted in center comes out clean.

Debbie Miller
Clarksdale

MICROWAVE SCALLOPED POTATOES

SERVES: 4 TO 6

4 medium potatoes
1 tablespoon all purpose
  flour
1 teaspoon salt

¼ cup chopped onion
½ cup milk
Butter or margarine

Peel and thinly slice potatoes. Arrange in a 3 quart glass casserole. Sprinkle on flour, salt and chopped onion. Pour milk over all. Dot with margarine. Cover with glass lid or plastic wrap. Microwave on high for 10 minutes. Stir and recover, cooking on high for 8 to 10 minutes or until potatoes are tender. Let stand 5 minutes before serving.

Rita Moser
Clarksdale

SCALLOPED POTATOES

SERVES: 6 TO 8   OVEN: 350°

8 cups peeled, thinly sliced
  potatoes (4 to 6 potatoes)
6 hard cooked eggs, sliced
1½ cups chopped green
  onions

¼ cup melted margarine
2 teaspoons salt
½ teaspoon pepper
1½ cups half and half

Combine all ingredients except half and half in a 3 quart casserole. Pour half and half over slowly. Bake 1 to 1½ hours or until potatoes are tender.

Georgia Haaga
Clarksdale

SPICY ITALIAN POTATOES

SERVES: 4 TO 6   OVEN: 350°

4 or 5 medium to large
  potatoes
¾ cup margarine

1 package dry Italian salad
  dressing mix

Peel and quarter potatoes. Boil 5 minutes and drain. Melt margarine and mix with dry salad dressing mix. Pour over potatoes and bake uncovered for about 30 minutes.

Regina Williams
Rome

BAKED SPINACH

SERVES: 8   OVEN: 325°

2 (10 ounce) packages frozen
  chopped spinach
4 tablespoons butter
½ cup chopped onion
½ cup chopped celery
½ pound fresh mushrooms,
  or 1 (4 ounce) can sliced
5 eggs
½ cup extra fine bread
  crumbs

1 (10¾ ounce) can cream of
  mushroom soup
1 (8 ounce) carton cottage
  cheese
⅛ teaspoon oregano
½ teaspoon pepper
¼ cup grated Parmesan
  cheese

Pour hot water over spinach to thaw; or remove from freezer and put in refrigerator the day before to let it thaw. Strain raw spinach, making sure all water is pressed out. Melt butter. Sauté onion, celery, and mushrooms until onion is opaque. Beat eggs. Combine with crumbs, soup, cottage cheese, seasonings, and spinach. Mix with onion mixture. Pour into greased 9 inch square pan and sprinkle top with Parmesan cheese. Bake for 30 minutes. Cool. Cut in 1 inch squares or serve warm in larger squares as a luncheon vegetable.

Yvonne Rossie Abraham
Clarksdale

FRITTATA (SPINACH WITH EGGS)

SERVES: 4

1 garlic bud
2 tablespoons olive oil
2 tablespoons butter
2 (10 ounce) packages frozen
  spinach, cooked and
  drained well

Salt and pepper to taste
3 eggs, beaten
3 tablespoons Parmesan
  cheese

Mash a garlic bud and brown in olive oil and butter. Remove garlic from skillet. Add 2 packages spinach. Steam slowly for ten minutes. Add salt and pepper to taste. Pour eggs and Parmesan cheese over spinach. Cook over low heat without further stirring until eggs are set.

Toni M. Hardin
Duncan

SPANOCCOPETA (SPINACH PETA)

SERVES: 12   OVEN: 450°

3 pounds fresh spinach or 5
(10 ounce) boxes frozen
spinach
3 bunches fresh green
onions, chopped
2 tablespoons dry dillweed
1 bunch chopped parsley
7 to 8 well beaten eggs
1 tablespoon farina (or cream
of wheat)

½ pound crumbled feta
cheese
¼ cup grated Parmesan
cheese
¼ cup olive oil
Salt to taste
1½ cups margarine, melted
1 pound filo

Wash spinach and drain well (if using frozen spinach, thaw overnight and press out all water). Sprinkle with salt. Combine with onions, dill, parsley, farina, cheeses, oil and eggs. Line an 11 x 5 x 2 inch pan with 8 filo leaves, brushing with melted butter between each layer. Pour in spinach mixture. Cover with 8 more filo leaves brushing each with butter. Brush tip with butter and sprinkle lightly with water. Bake for 15 to 20 minutes until filo begins to turn a light golden color and puffs in the center. Reduce oven to 350° and bake 30 minutes longer until golden brown. Let peta stand 15 to 20 minutes before cutting.

Helen Valsamakis
Clarksdale

FORGOTTEN SQUASH

SERVES: 6

4 medium size yellow
squash, split

4 tablespoons margarine
Salt and pepper to taste

Wash and dry squash; split lengthwise. Place in a microwave-safe baking dish and cover with plastic wrap if dish does not have a top. This is the crazy part - bake on high 10 minutes. Pour off excess liquid and bake 5 minutes longer. Drain again. Uncover squash and bake 5 more minutes. The squash will dehydrate. Top each with a pat of margarine and sprinkle with salt and pepper. Cook on high 5 minutes more. The results are a chewy, nutty tasting squash. It makes a good finger food for children.

Roselyn B. Dulaney
Clarksdale

BOOGA BOTTOM TURNIP GREENS

You have got to wash them real good, 6 or 7 times. Tear the stems out of the leaves and tear the leaves. Put them in a pot and bring to a boil. Pour this water off and start over. You use enough water to cover the greens. If you have three bunches of greens, use about a quart of water. In the second cooking: add salt meat to the bottom of the pot (can substitute bacon slices). Cut up your salt meat into 1 inch pieces. Use about 6 one inch pieces. If you use salt meat you do not add salt. If you use bacon, add 1 teaspoon salt and 2 tablespoons sugar. Put your greens in the pot and add enough water to cover, about 2 cups. Bring back to boil and simmer for at least 30 minutes. Always cover the pot on the last cooking.

Family Secret: This method is also used on mustard greens and collards. You do add more sugar to collards, about another tablespoon. Also this is the way Mildred cooks cabbage. She does cut down her water to one cup on the second cooking of cabbage.

Mildred Burkes
Duncan

SQUASH CASSEROLE

SERVES: 6 TO 8   OVEN: 325°

6 medium yellow squash
1 medium onion, diced
1 cup water
½ teaspoon salt
½ teaspoon pepper
2 eggs, beaten
¼ pound cheese

¼ cup milk (sweet)
1 (16 ounce) can tomatoes,
   drained (optional)
1½ cups cracker crumbs
   (soda)
⅓ stick of margarine

Cut squash into halves. Add onion, water, and salt and pepper. Cover and cook until tender. Drain off all water. Add beaten eggs, milk, cheese, and tomatoes (optional). Put squash mixture in baking dish (8 inch square or equal size) and top with crushed soda crackers. Dot top with slivers of margarine. Bake approximately 25 minutes until top is brown and casserole is set firm.

Margarite Harris
"Booga Bottom"
Duncan

STUFFED SQUASH

YIELD: 6 TO 8

8 medium-sized yellow
squash, room temperature
1 pound ground beef or
chuck
¾ cup uncooked rice
½ cup scooped squash
1 (16 ounce can) whole
tomatoes

1 can water
1 teaspoon salt
1 teaspoon black pepper
¾ teaspoon ground cinnamon
1 tablespoon lemon juice

Wash squash. Cut off enough on rounded end to allow for scooping. Save tip. Scoop out squash, leaving about ¼ inch thickness. (If regular scooper not available, use potato peeler and scooper.) Rinse squash. Combine meat, rice, scooped squash, the whole tomatoes (reserving liquid for later use), salt, pepper, and cinnamon. Mix thoroughly, mashing tomatoes well. Stuff squash loosely, about ¾ full. (If packed too tight, squash will burst, as rice must have room to swell.) Place squash in boiler; add cut-off tips and reserved tomato juice, plus 1 can of water. Simmer 30 minutes. Add lemon juice and cook 15 minutes longer.

Family Secret: You may prefer cutting off the neck of squash and scooping from there. Tiny eggplant, zucchini, or bell peppers may be used as squash substitute.

Yvonne Rossie Abraham
Clarksdale

ITALIAN ZUCCHINI CRESCENT PIE

SERVES: 6 TO 8

OVEN: 375°

4 cups thinly sliced zucchini
1 cup chopped onion
¼ to ½ cup margarine or
butter
½ cup chopped parsley or 2
tablespoons parsley flakes
½ teaspoon salt
½ teaspoon pepper
¼ teaspoon garlic powder

¼ teaspoon basil
¼ teaspoon oregano
1 8 ounce can crescent dinner
rolls
2 teaspoons mustard
2 beaten eggs
2 cups mozzarella or
muenster cheese, shredded
(8 ounces)

VEGETABLES

CONTINUED, ITALIAN ZUCCHINI CRESCENT PIE

Cook and stir zucchini and onion in melted butter in large skillet.
Cook for 5 minutes then add parsley, salt, pepper, garlic, basil, and
oregano. Remove from heat. In 9 inch or 10 inch ungreased pie pan
press crescent rolls that have been separated first into triangles.
Using fingers, press over bottom and up sides to form crust. Spread
crust with mustard. Add eggs and cheese to slightly cooled zucchini
mixture. Pour vegetable mixture into crust. Bake until center is set.
Cover crust with foil during last 10 minutes of baking. Let stand 10
minutes before serving. You may bake and reheat in microwave.

Family Secret: Even people that have never liked zucchini have
enjoyed it prepared like this. My kids love it and call it "zucchini
pizza"!

Sara Lynn Masey
Marks

MRS. CADE'S VEGETABLE PIE

SERVES: 8   OVEN: 400°

3 tablespoons butter or   1 diced tomato
  margarine   Pinch of basil
1 large onion, chopped   2 tablespoons sugar
1 cup chopped mushrooms   Salt and pepper to taste
1 bell pepper, chopped   9 inch pie shell
1 large squash, diced   1 cup mayonnaise
1 large zucchini, diced   1 cup mozzarella cheese

Sauté onions, mushrooms, and bell pepper. Set aside. Boil squash
and zucchini until tender and then drain. Mix above two together.
Add tomato, sugar, salt, pepper, and basil. Cook all for 10 minutes.
Drain. Bake pie shell for 10 minutes. Pour all in pie shell. Mix cheese
and mayonnaise together and put on top. Bake for 10 minutes at
400° to brown top, then 50 minutes at 350° covered. Spray cooking
spray on foil so it will not stick to cheese and mayonnaise top.

Chris Heaton
Clarksdale

Health Secret: Beta - carotene has been shown to lower cancer
risk. Our daily need is fulfilled by eating several of the following:
1 sweet potato, 1 cup spinach or collard greens, 1 medium carrot,
½ cantaloupe, 3 stalks broccoli, 6 small apricots.

BÉARNAISE SAUCE

YIELD: ½ TO ¾ CUP

2 egg yolks
1 stick hot melted butter
1 tablespoon tarragon
  vinegar

Salt and red pepper to taste
2 tablespoons chopped
  chives (add after making)

Blend eggs, salt, pepper, and vinegar in blender. While blender is running, add hot butter in a steady stream. Add chives.

Family Secret: Serve with Beef Tenderloin.

Nancy Easley
Clarksdale

HOMEMADE MAYONNAISE

YIELD: 1 PINT

2 egg yolks
2 cups oil
Juice of 1 to 2 lemons

½ teaspoon salt
¼ teaspoon red pepper

It is very important to add oil to egg yolks slowly. Put egg yolks in smaller electric beater bowl. Have ready juice of lemons with salt and pepper. Measure oil. Start beating egg yolks and gradually add oil, drop by drop, at first until eggs thicken. If you add oil too fast, it will go back to oil. As mixture thickens, you can add oil faster. Also add lemon juice to egg mixture as needed to thin mayonnaise to desired consistency. Refrigerate.

Florence Larson
Friars Point

SAL'S RELISH FOR STRING BEANS

1 pound can beets, drained
  and chopped
½ cup chopped celery
½ cup chopped bell pepper
2 medium onions, chopped

½ tablespoon of
  Worcestershire sauce
2 tablespoons of catsup
1 cup mayonnaise
Salt to taste

Mix all ingredients, chill, and serve over hot fresh string beans.

Mrs. Bill Luckett
Clarksdale

REMOULADE SAUCE FOR SHRIMP

YIELD: 2 PINTS

2 hard boiled eggs, grated
2 branches celery, chopped
 fine
1 tablespoon Worcestershire
 sauce
3 tablespoons dry mustard

8 tablespoons Creole mus-
 tard
1 teaspoon salt
1 teaspoon sugar
1 pint mayonnaise
1 garlic clove, crushed

Mix all ingredients.

Maggie Sherard
Sherard

MARINARA SAUCE

This simple tomato sauce arrived from the Italian Delta of Bologna. Preferably, use fresh delta-raised Italian plum tomatoes. If not available, use canned plum tomatoes.

2¼ pounds fresh plum
 tomatoes
1 medium yellow onion,
 peeled and slashed (on
 bottom)

1 teaspoon salt
¼ teaspoon sugar
¼ pound butter

Put tomatoes in boiling water long enough for skins to pop. Drain and peel. Purée in food processor. Put tomatoes in pot (uncovered) with onion, salt, sugar, and butter. Simmer 1 hour. Save onion for soup or eat with butter. If preparing this sauce for the freezer, hold the butter. Add when heating to use.

Family Secret: We use it on pasta, fried eggplant, fried green tomatoes, pork chops - really most anything. A son-in-law says it would be good on ice cream.

The Phantom of the Delta - Lowell Taylor
Hughes, Arkansas

CHILI SAUCE

YIELD: 16 PINT JARS

2 gallons chopped tomatoes
(skin first, hot water
method)
1 quart chopped onions
10 to 15 small hot peppers

As many green bell peppers
as you prefer, chopped
½ teaspoon ground cloves
½ teaspoon ground allspice
½ cup salt, plain not iodized

Mix all this together and boil slowly about 1½ hours or until thick - then add:

3½ cups cider vinegar
5 cups sugar

1 teaspoon cinnamon
2 tablespoons chili powder

Continue boiling for 20 minutes - then spoon into canning jars and seal immediately. Process in boiling water bath for 15 minutes.

Family Secret: Will be thick and good!

Mrs. Felix West
Clarksdale

"BUN-YUT"

YIELD: ABOUT 1½ CUPS

Bunch of parsley
3 to 4 garlic buds
¾ cup oil

¼ cup vinegar
Dash hot sauce

Chop parsley and garlic. Add oil and vinegar as proportioned above. Add dash of hot sauce. Place in tightly covered jar. Let stand a day or two before eating. Refrigerate.

Family Secret: This relish is used as an accompaniment to meat and is called in dialect "Bun-Yut." (Phonetic spelling - there is not "uh" sound in pure Italian.) Probably derives from "Bagna-Cauda" meaning "Hot Bath" or dip.

Perian Conerly
Clarksdale

BUTLER RELISH

YIELD: APPROXIMATELY 4 CUPS

4 tomatoes, chopped
1 bell pepper, chopped
1 onion, chopped
Salt and pepper (⅛ teaspoon each)

⅓ cup vinegar
1 tablespoon of sugar

Peel and cut tomatoes in small pieces. Mix and toss.

Family Secret: Use as a condiment.

Barbara Graves
Clarksdale

TOMATO GRAVY

1 tablespoon shortening (not oil)
2 tablespoons flour (maybe more - will know when cooking)
1 large glass water (about 1½ cups)

1 (10 ounce) can stewed tomatoes or 9 ripe tomatoes, chopped
Salt and pepper to taste

Melt shortening in 10½ inch iron skillet; when hot add flour (must be thick). Brown flour till dark in color. Mix half the water with tomatoes and add to brown flour. Stir while pouring. Then add remaining water until medium thickness. Add salt and pepper.

Family Secret: Serve over biscuits, alone, or with bacon, sausage, and eggs. This is great for a breakfast dish on a cold morning and really fills the kids up.

Mrs. Joy Wilkerson
Lambert

MINT PEPPER JELLY

YIELD: 6 HALF PINTS

2 cups fresh-picked mint,
  packed
3¼ cups water
Green food coloring
½ teaspoon fresh lemon juice

1 (1¾ ounce) box commercial
  pectin
4 cups sugar
6 hot peppers, cut fine

In 4 quart boiler put crushed mint and stems and water; bring to a boil. Remove from heat, cover and let stand ten minutes. Strain and measure 3 cups of mint infusion. Add food coloring and lemon juice. Add commercial pectin, dissolve and bring to a boil rapidly. Add sugar and hot peppers and cook fast, stirring until it comes to a rapid boil that cannot be stirred down; then cook one minute more. Pour into sterilized jelly glasses and seal.

Family Secret: Very nice served with lamb and ham. Also good served over cream cheese with crackers. I prepare recipe to 3 cups infusion. Cool and place in freezer container while mint is in peak of growth and freeze. When peppers reach their bright red color of peak flavor I remove infusion and complete recipe.

Jewell Graeber

BELL PEPPER RELISH

YIELD: 8 PINTS

12 red peppers
12 green peppers
12 onions
2 cups vinegar

2 cups sugar
1 to 3 tablespoons salt
(Add 1 hot pepper, if desired)

Chop peppers and onions. Cover with boiling water and let stand 5 minutes. Drain well. Put vegetables into large pan. Add vinegar, sugar, and salt. Boil 5 minutes. Pour into sterilized pint jars and seal in boiling water bath for 15 minutes.

Family Secret: Gives a great "zip" to field peas and butter beans.

Emily Cooper
Clarksdale

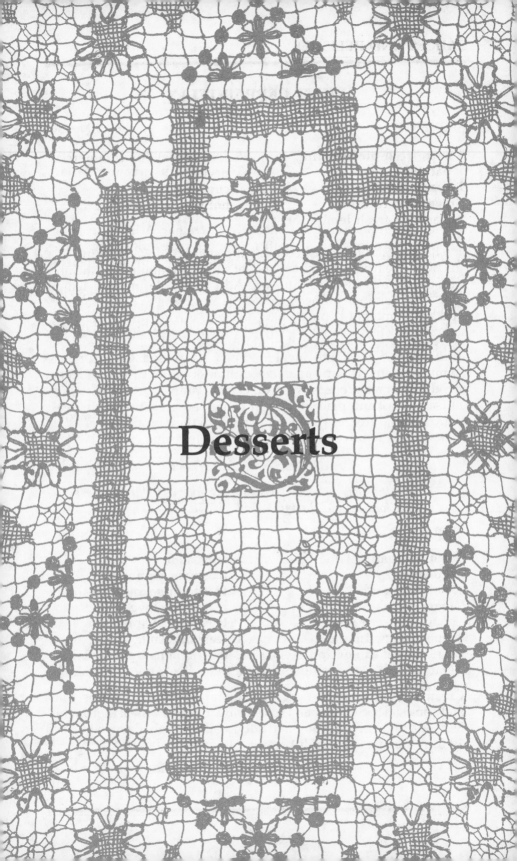

Desserts

ANGEL FOOD CAKE

SERVES: 12   OVEN: 350°

1 cup sifted cake flour
1½ cups sifted sugar
1¼ cups egg whites (9 to 11 eggs)

¼ teaspoon salt
1¼ teaspoons cream of tartar

Sift cake flour once and then measure. Sift sugar. Add ½ cup of the sugar to the cake flour and sift four more times. Beat egg whites with salt with wire whisk and beat until foamy. Sprinkle in cream of tartar and beat until it stands in peaks but not dry. It should be soft and glassy. Sprinkle the rest of the sugar (1 cup) over egg whites, 4 tablespoons at a time. Beat 10 strokes after each addition. Sprinkle ¼ of flour mixture and beat 15 times turning bowl lightly. For good luck, fold 10 strokes more. Add flour mixture as above until all gone. Turn into angel food pan, ungreased. Cook for 30 to 35 minutes. Invert pan and balance on neck of soft drink bottle. Let stand 1 hour before removing cake from pan.

Darbra McDowell Holcomb
Duncan

APPLESAUCE CAKE

My mother had a knack for whipping up good things to eat despite food rations during World War II.

SERVES: 12   OVEN: 350°

⅔ cup margarine (10⅔ table-spoons)
1½ cups sugar
2 eggs
½ pound box of raisins
1 cup chopped pecans
1 (15 ounce) can of apple-sauce

3 cups flour
1 teaspoon cinnamon
½ teaspoon nutmeg
½ teaspoon cloves
½ teaspoon allspice
1 teaspoon soda
2 tablespoons boiling water

Cream margarine and sugar. Add eggs and beat. Add raisins, nuts, and applesauce. Sift flour and spices. Add to mixture. Beat thoroughly. Stir soda into boiling water and add to cake dough. Bake in greased 10 inch tube pan or bundt pan for 1 hour and 20 minutes.

Mrs T. J. Cassidy, Jr.
Lula

JIMMIE LOU'S GREEN APPLE CAKE

SERVES: 10 TO 12 OVEN: 350°

2 cups sugar
4 eggs, well beaten
3 cups flour
2 teaspoons baking powder
1 teaspoon baking soda
1 teaspoon salt
½ teaspoon nutmeg
½ teaspoon ground cloves

½ teaspoon allspice
2 teaspoons cinnamon
½ cup strong cool liquid
   coffee
1½ cups cooking oil
1 cup raisins
3 cups raw green apples,
   chopped

Mix together sugar and eggs and beat until light and fluffy. Sift dry ingredients. Combine coffee and oil and add to first mixture alternating with dry ingredients. Add raisins and apples. Bake in greased tube pan for one to one and a half hours.

Family Secret: Stays moist forever.

Mrs. Gus Brown, Jr. (Emma)
Marks

Mrs.Jeff Clark
Clarksdale

COCONUT POUND CAKE

SERVES: 10 TO 12 COLD OVEN

1 cup vegetable shortening
½ cup margarine, softened
3 cups sugar
6 eggs
1 teaspoon coconut extract

1 teaspoon almond extract
3 cups cake flour
1 cup milk
1 (7 ounce) can coconut

Cream shortening and margarine. Add sugar very slowly. Add eggs one at a time, beating one minute between each. Add extract, then flour and milk alternately, beginning and ending with milk. (Be sure to do this very slowly. It takes about 10 minutes.) Add coconut and mix well. Pour in a well greased and floured tube pan. Put in cold oven. Turn oven to 300° and bake for 1½ to 2 hours.

Family Secret: This is my brother's favorite!

Gayla Marley
Clarksdale

BANANA SPICE CAKE
WITH SEA-FOAM ICING

SERVES: 12 TO 16   OVEN: 350°

CAKE:

2½ cups sifted cake flour
1⅔ cups sugar
1¼ teaspoons baking powder
1¼ teaspoons baking soda
1 teaspoon salt
1½ teaspoons cinnamon
¾ teaspoon nutmeg

½ teaspoon ground cloves
⅔ cup vegetable shortening
⅔ cup buttermilk
1¼ cups mashed ripe bananas
  (about 3 medium)
2 eggs, unbeaten

Sift dry ingredients into large mixer bowl. Add shortening, buttermilk, and mashed bananas. Mix until all flour is dampened. Beat at low speed for 2 minutes. Add eggs. Beat 1 minute. Turn batter into three 8 inch or two 9 inch greased and floured cake pans. Bake for 30 to 35 minutes or until cake springs when lightly touched.

SEA-FOAM ICING:

2 egg whites
1½ cups light brown sugar
  (firmly packed)
5 tablespoons water
Dash of salt

1 teaspoon vanilla
2 squares sweet cooking
  chocolate
1 tablespoon butter

Combine egg whites, sugar, water, and salt in top of double boiler. Beat slightly to mix. Place over rapidly boiling water. Beat with rotary egg beater or electric mixer at high speed until frosting stands in peaks, about 7 minutes. Remove from heat. Add vanilla. Beat 1 to 2 more minutes or until thick enough to spread. Spread Sea-Foam Icing between cooled layers. Make swirls on top and spoon melted chocolate into swirls. For swirls: Melt chocolate and butter together. Mix well and cool. For lots of frosting, double the recipe.

Mrs. Felix West
Clarksdale

CARROT CAKE

SERVES: 10 TO 12   OVEN: 350°

4 eggs
2½ cups flour (plain)
2 tablespoons wheat germ
2 cups sugar
2 teaspoons cinnamon

2 teaspoons baking soda
1 teaspoon salt
1½ cups vegetable oil
3 jars strained carrots
1 cup pecans

CONTINUED, CARROT CAKE

Beat eggs. Add remaining ingredients. Mix well at low speed of electric mixer. Pour into two greased and floured 8 inch cake pans. Bake for 30 to 35 minutes or until cake tester comes out clean.

CREAM CHEESE FROSTING:
1 (8 ounce) package cream cheese, softened
½ cup butter, softened

1 (1 pound) box powdered sugar
1 teaspoon vanilla

Beat well. Spread on cool cake. Top with pecans.

Susan B. Houston
Clarksdale

SWEET POTATO CAKE:
Substitute 1½ cups grated raw sweet potatoes for carrots.

Mary McClain
Clarksdale

CHEESECAKE FOR 30 (INDIVIDUAL)

YIELD: 30   OVEN: 350°

CAKE:
3 (8 ounce) packages cream cheese, softened
5 eggs
1 cup sugar

1½ teaspoons vanilla
1 bag (good) vanilla wafers
Cupcake liners, or cups - (foil)

Cream softened cream cheese, eggs, sugar, and vanilla. Place wafer flat side down in each cupcake cup. Fill ¾ full and bake 20 minutes. Cool 5 minutes.

TOPPING:
¼ cup sour cream
⅓ cup sugar

1 teaspoon vanilla

Combine topping ingredients and put 1 teaspoon on each cheesecake. Bake 5 minutes more.

Family Secret: Can use cherry pie filling to top. Can add 1 tablespoon lemon juice to sour cream mixture.

Sheila Roberts
Clarksdale

CHEESE CAKE

SERVES: 16   OVEN: 350°

CRUST:
1½ cups graham cracker   ¼ cup powdered sugar
  crumbs (about 20 crackers)   ½ cup melted butter

Lightly oil bottom of springform pan. Combine crumbs, powdered sugar and butter for crust until thoroughly mixed. Press into bottom of springform pan. Bake 5 minutes in preheated oven. Place on rack to cool.

FILLING:
4 (8 ounce) packages cream   1 teaspoon vanilla
  cheese, softened   6 eggs
1 cup granulated sugar

Cream the cheese until light. Add sugar and vanilla and cream again. Add eggs one at a time, beating well after each. Pour over cooled crust and bake 40 minutes. Cool 15 minutes on rack.

TOPPING:
2 cups sour cream   1 teaspoon vanilla
1⅓ cups powdered sugar   Cinnamon

Thoroughly mix sour cream, powdered sugar and vanilla. Pour carefully over baked cheese cake. Sprinkle with generous amount of cinnamon. Bake 10 minutes Cool to room temperature and then chill 12 to 24 hours before serving. Remove side piece from pan and cut into wedges.

Mrs. Elzy J. Smith
Clarksdale

HARVEY'S LEMON CHEESE CAKE

SERVES: 12   OVEN: 350°

CRUST:
2 cups graham cracker   ¼ cup sugar
  crumbs   ½ cup margarine (melted)

Combine all 3 ingredients. Press on bottom and sides of 9 inch spring pan. Bake 8 to 10 minutes.

CONTINUED, HARVEY'S LEMON CHEESE CAKE

FILLING:

4 medium eggs - separated	1 cup sour cream
⅛ teaspoon salt	⅓ cup lemon juice
3 (8 ounce) packages cream cheese, softened	2 tablespoons flour
	1 cup whipped cream
2 cups sugar	

Reduce oven temperature to 325°. Beat egg whites with salt and set aside (if you use large eggs the cake will be too big for the pan.) Cream the cream cheese and sugar, then beat several minutes with mixer on high. Blend in egg yolks, one at a time, then sour cream and lemon juice. Add flour. Beat all together on medium high setting for several minutes. Fold in egg whites. Pour into crust and bake 1 hour and 15 minutes at 325°. Open oven door slightly and leave cake in oven to cool. Refrigerate and when cold top with whipped cream.

Harvey Fiser
Clarksdale

CIVIL WAR CAKE

A freed slave taught her former mistress to bake this cake. Mother passed the recipe to daughter by word of mouth until recent times when it was written down by Eunice Phillips Clark.

OVEN: 375°

1 cup sugar	3 teaspoons baking powder
½ cup shortening	½ teaspoon salt
1 teaspoon vanilla	8 ounces dried apples
½ cup milk	¾ cup sugar
1 egg	Water
2½ cups flour	

Cream together sugar, shortening, and vanilla. Add egg and milk and mix well. Add flour, salt, and baking powder. Divide into 4 or 5 parts, shape into balls, roll out thin (like cookie dough) to size of a plate. Bake on cookie sheet until light brown. Put dried apples in pan and cover with water. When almost done, sweeten with ¾ cup sugar, mash with potato masher (If too runny, pour off some liquid). Allow apples to cool before stacking cake layers with apples between each layer. Don't put apples on top. Just before serving, sprinkle a little granulated sugar on top. Best if cooked the day before serving. Trim cake to an even round shape as you are cutting it to serve.

Jean Duff
Alligator

DATE NUT CAKE

SERVES: 30   OVEN: 275° TO 300°

1 cup butter, softened
2 cups sugar
½ cup white corn syrup
6 whole eggs
4 cups plain flour, sifted
(save ½ cup for fruit and
nuts)
1 whole grated nutmeg or 2
teaspoons ground nutmeg

2 teaspoons baking powder
½ cup whiskey (divided)
1 pound pitted dates
1 cup raisins
1 quart (4 cups) pecan pieces
¼ cup port wine

Cream butter and sugar in large mixing bowl. Add syrup then eggs, one at a time. Sift flour, nutmeg, and baking powder. Combine with butter mixture, alternating with ¼ cup whiskey. Dust fruit and nuts with ½ cup flour; add to mixture. Grease 3 large loaf pans, then line them with wax paper. Put cake in pans. Place pans in a shallow pan of water in oven. Bake about 3 hours. When cake is done peel paper off while still hot. Put cakes back in pans and pour over them a mixture of ¼ cup whiskey and ¼ cup port wine. When cool, wrap in foil and store in a cool closet. Pour a little whiskey over cakes every 2 weeks until the cake is eaten. (Does not freeze well.)

Patsy Maclin
Clarksdale

CHOCOLATE ICE BOX CAKE

SERVES: 8

1 dozen macaroons
2 to 3 tablespoons sherry
1 dozen lady fingers, split
2 squares bitter chocolate
½ cup strong coffee
¾ cup granulated sugar

4 eggs, separated
2 sticks butter, softened
1 cup powdered sugar
1 cup pecans, chopped
1 teaspoon vanilla

Crumble macaroons and dribble sherry to moisten; put in bottom of 2-quart springform pan; line sides of pan with lady fingers. Melt chocolate; add coffee, granulated sugar, and egg yolks; mix well. Cream butter and powdered sugar; add chocolate mixture. Beat egg whites until stiff; fold into mixture. Add pecans and vanilla. Pour into springform pan and refrigerate until time to serve.

Barbara Mullins
Clarksdale

MISS MINNIE'S CHOCOLATE FUDGE CAKE

SERVES 12 TO 15   OVEN: 350°

CAKE:

2 sticks margarine or butter	1½ cups plain flour
2 cups sugar	1 teaspoon vanilla extract
4 eggs	2 cups miniature
4 tablespoons cocoa	marshmallows

Cream butter, add sugar and cream. Add eggs and beat well. Sift cocoa and flour and add to mixture. Add vanilla and pour into greased 13 x 9 x 2 inch baking pan. Bake for 35 minutes. Remove from oven and place two cups (or more) miniature marshmallows on top of cake. Return to oven to melt (about 2 to 3 minutes).

FROSTING:

1 stick margarine or butter	6 ounce package semi-sweet
2 cups sugar	chocolate chips
¾ cup evaporated milk	1 teaspoon vanilla extract
2 cups miniature	
marshmallows	

Boil margarine, milk and sugar, stirring constantly for nine minutes. Remove from heat, add marshmallows and chocolate chips and stir until melted. Add vanilla and cool. Spread over cake in the pan. Let cool two hours or overnight before cutting.

Nancy M. Daughdrill
Clarksdale

FUDGE CAKE

SERVES: 10 TO 20   OVEN: 300°

½ cup butter, softened	½ teaspoon baking powder
2 cups sugar	4 tablespoons cocoa
3 eggs	1 cup chopped pecans
1 cup sifted flour	1 teaspoon vanilla
¼ teaspoon salt	1 tablespoon milk

Cream butter and sugar. Add eggs one at a time. Sift dry ingredients. Combine milk and vanilla. Alternately add milk mixture and dry ingredients to butter and eggs. Fold in pecans. Pour into greased and floured 11¾ x 7½ inch pan. Bake for 1 hour. Cut into squares when cool. Be sure not to over-bake. You want these to be chewy.

Laurenze Cooper Bouldin (Mrs. Marshall Bouldin, Sr.)
Clarksdale

HONEY'S FRUIT CAKE

About two weeks before every Christmas the aroma of Honey's Fruit Cake initiated the holiday season. Mama made 1 large cake for Christmas dinner and a small cake that was always left by the fireplace for Santa.

SERVES: 15 TO 18   OVEN: 250°

½ pound butter, softened
2 cups sugar
10 eggs, separated
½ cup whiskey
Juice of coconut
3 cups flour
1½ teaspoons cinnamon
½ teaspoon allspice
½ teaspoon cloves

1 coconut, drained and grated
4 pounds candied pineapple
½ pound blanched almonds
2 pounds candied cherries
1 pound candied citron
¼ pound candied lemon
1½ quarts pecans

Cream softened butter and sugar (saving out ½ cup of sugar). Add egg yolks, then liquids, constantly beating. Sift together flour and spices. Cut cherries and pineapple into small pieces. Mix all fruits and nuts with flour mixture. Use hands to mix so that fruit is coated and separated. Grease tube pan and line with brown paper that is also lightly greased. Add butter mixture to fruit. Beat egg whites slowly adding the last ½ cup of sugar. Mix this mixture into fruit mixture. Put in pans. On a low rack, put a cake pan filled with water. Put tube pans on the middle rack in oven. Steam cakes for about 3 or 4 hours.

Kay Allen
Clarksdale

SOFT GINGER BREAD

SERVES: 8 TO 10   OVEN: 350°

2 teaspoons baking soda
1¼ cups buttermilk
1 cup molasses
¾ cup butter or margarine, melted
2¼ cups all-purpose flour, unsifted

1 cup sugar, white or light brown
3 teaspoons ground ginger
½ teaspoon salt
3 eggs
¼ teaspoon vanilla
1 cup raisins or chopped nuts

Put soda in buttermilk. Add molasses and melted margarine and stir well. Sift dry ingredients and add to the liquids. Beat vigorously. Add eggs one at a time, beating well with each addition. Add vanilla and stir in raisins or nuts. Pour into a well greased and floured 9 inch x 13 inch pan. Bake in oven for 45 to 50 minutes.

CONTINUED, SOFT GINGER BREAD

HARD SAUCE:
4 tablespoons soft margarine   Pinch salt
  (or more)   Juice of 1 large lemon
1 tablespoon boiling water
1 cup confectioner's sugar,
  sifted

Beat margarine until fluffy. Add sugar, a small amount at a time.
Add boiling water, salt and lemon juice. Spoon on warm ginger
bread. Serve warm.

Family Secret: This is my mother's German recipe and is over 100
years old.

Hazel Boyd
Clarksdale

GLADYS TIPLER'S LEMON CREAM CAKE

SERVES: 12 TO 14   OVEN: 350°

3 half pints whipping cream   1½ cups powdered sugar,
2 (3 ounce) boxes lemon   sifted
  gelatin   Juice of 1 lemon
1 box yellow cake mix, sifted

The night before you bake, stir together the whipping cream and
gelatin. Do not whip, just stir in. Put this in a large bowl, cover and
refrigerate. Sift cake mix and follow directions on box for baking in
2 round layers. (Sifting the cake mix makes a lighter cake.) When
layers are completely cool, split them with a very sharp knife to
make 4 layers. Whip the cream and gelatin mixture until stiff. Add
the powdered sugar and the lemon juice. Spread generously between
layers, on top and sides of cake. To freeze: Freeze before wrapping
so the wrapping won't stick to the filling. When completely frozen,
cover. This will keep for weeks in the freezer. Especially suited for
a ladies' party.

Mrs. Rick Parsons
Clarksdale

JAMEYE BARNES' MAHOGANY CAKE

Family Night Supper at the Presbyterian Church wasn't complete without Jameye's Mahogany Cake!

SERVES: 8 TO 10   OVEN: 325°

CAKE:

1 cup butter or margarine, softened	2 cups flour, sifted
1½ cups sugar	3 tablespoons cocoa
4 eggs, separated	1 teaspoon soda
1 teaspoon vanilla	1 cup buttermilk

Cream butter and sugar until light and fluffy; add well-beaten egg yolks and vanilla. Slow mixer to lowest speed; add sifted dry ingredients alternately with buttermilk. Fold in well-beaten egg whites. Bake for 25 minutes in two nine inch or ten inch pans.

ICING:

1 stick butter or margarine, softened	1 teaspoon vanilla
1 box powdered sugar	½ cup chopped pecans
1 egg	Grated rind of 1 small orange
2 tablespoons strong black coffee	Cream, if needed
2 squares melted un-sweetened chocolate	½ cup grated pecans

Place butter, sugar, egg, and coffee in mixing bowl and beat until light and fluffy; add melted chocolate, vanilla, nuts, grated rind. Add cream 1 tablespoon at a time (if needed) for right consistency. Ice cake. Garnish with ½ cup grated nuts on top of cake after icing.

Maggie Tyner
Clarksdale

MOM'S POUND CAKE

SERVES: 10 TO 12   OVEN: 325°

1 cup shortening less 1 tablespoon	1 tablespoon of grated lemon rind
3 cups sugar	1½ teaspoons vanilla
5 eggs	½ teaspoon lemon flavoring
3 cups flour	2 or 3 tablespoons of fresh lemon juice
½ teaspoon of soda dissolved in 1 cup buttermilk	

CONTINUED, MOM'S POUND CAKE

Cream shortening and sugar. Add egg yolks one at a time, beating well after each is added. Add flour alternately with buttermilk and soda mixture; add flavorings. Beat egg whites very stiff and fold into batter. Be sure egg whites and batter are well mixed, but do not beat. Bake in tube pan for 1 hour and 15 minutes.

Family Secret: It was my Grandmother's.

Merle Butler
Jonestown

MOTHER'S JAM CAKE

SERVES: 8 TO 10   OVEN: 350°

1½ cups butter, softened
2 cups sugar
3 cups jam, blueberry or
   blackberry
5 eggs, separated
4 cups of flour, sifted twice

1 cup buttermilk
1 teaspoon soda
2 teaspoons nutmeg
2 teaspoons ground cloves
2 teaspoons cinnamon
2 teaspoons allspice

Cream butter; add sugar and beat until light and fluffy. Add jam. Add well beaten egg yolks. Sift flour two or three times. Add the flour alternately with buttermilk, to which soda has been added. Add spices. Fold in egg whites, which have been beaten until stiff. Pour into two well greased 9 inch layer pan and bake for 35 to 40 minutes or until cake springs back when touched with your fingers.

BUTTERMILK CARAMEL ICING:
3 cups sugar, divided
3 tablespoons butter

1 cup buttermilk
¼ teaspoon soda

In an iron skillet cook ½ cup sugar to a golden brown syrup. Be careful you do not burn it. Warm milk to which soda has been added. Combine rest of sugar, butter and milk. Have the brown caramel syrup around the same temperature as the milk and soda and sugar and butter. Combine mixtures. Boil to a soft ball stage and let cool. Beat until icing turns light brown. Will frost a 2 layer cake.

Mrs. Gus Brown, Jr. (Emma)
Marks

HEATON'S TIPSY PECAN CAKE

SERVES: 10 TO 12   OVEN: 275°

¾ cup butter, softened
2¾ cups sugar
6 eggs, beaten separately
4 cups sifted flour

2 teaspoons nutmeg
4 cups chopped pecans
4½ cups raisins
½ cup whiskey

Cream butter, add sugar and egg yolks. Sift flour and nutmeg. Coat pecans and raisins with half of flour. Alternately add rest of flour with whiskey and beaten egg whites to butter mixture. Add pecans and raisins. Pour into greased bundt pan. Bake 2 hours.

Chris Heaton
Clarksdale

PRUNE CAKE

SERVES: 10 TO 12   CAKE: 350°

CAKE:
1 cup vegetable oil
1½ cups sugar
3 eggs
2 cups flour
1 teaspoon salt
1 teaspoon baking soda
1 teaspoon baking powder

1 teaspoon cinnamon
1 teaspoon nutmeg
1 teaspoon allspice
1 cup buttermilk
1 cup seeded, chopped
prunes
1 teaspoon vanilla

Cream oil and sugar together. Add eggs; mix well. Sift dry ingredients. Add buttermilk alternately with dry ingredients. Add prunes and vanilla. Pour into three 8-inch cake pans. Bake 20-25 minutes.

CUSTARD FILLING:
3 tablespoons cornstarch
1 cup sugar
3 eggs

2 cups scalded milk
½ cup butter or margarine
1 teaspoon vanilla

Mix cornstarch, sugar, eggs and milk together in top of double boiler. Cook until thick. Add butter and vanilla. Mix well. Let cool then chill in refrigerator. Divide custard between cake layers. Ice with favorite caramel icing.

Matsy Shea
Dumas, Arkansas

GERMAN CRUMB CAKE

SERVES: 24   OVEN: 350°

2 cups brown sugar (1 pound   1 teaspoon soda
  box)   2 teaspoons nutmeg
2 cups all-purpose flour   2 teaspoons cinnamon
1 cup butter or margarine   2 eggs
  (2 sticks)   1 cup buttermilk

Mix sugar with flour; then cut in butter with knives until mixture is crumbly, the size of small peas. Reserve 1 cup of mixture. Add soda and spices to remaining mixture. Add unbeaten eggs to buttermilk and mix slightly. Add to dry mixture. Pour into 2 greased and floured cake pans or one 13 x 9 inch pan. Sprinkle the cup of reserved mixture over the top. Bake for about 25 to 30 minutes.

Family Secret: This recipe has been in the family for three generations.

Shirley Easley
Clarksdale

OLD FASHIONED YELLOW CAKE

This recipe has been handed down for 4 generations in my mother's family.

SERVES: 12 TO 15   OVEN: 350°

1 cup of butter, softened   3½ level teaspoons baking
2 cups of sugar   powder
6 whole eggs   1 teaspoon vanilla
3½ cups sifted flour   1 cup sweet milk (whole)

Cream butter and sugar thoroughly. Add eggs one at a time, beating after each addition. Sift flour and baking powder. Add dry ingredients alternately with milk. Add vanilla. Bake in three layers for 20 to 25 minutes.

Fran Mullens
Lyon

APPLE PIE

SERVES: 8 - 10   OVEN: 325°

9 medium apples, peeled and   ½ cup brown sugar
  cored   ½ teaspoon cinnamon
2 teaspoons lemon juice   1 double pie crust recipe
½ cup sugar   ⅓ stick margarine

I use firm apples. Put apples in food processor with chopping blade. Pulse chop for about 6 seconds. Turn chopped apples into large mixing bowl. Add lemon juice, mix well. Add ½ cup sugar and ½ cup brown sugar. Mix well. Sprinkle with cinnamon. Pour apples into unbaked pie shell and top with slices of margarine. (This is a big mound of apples. Use the largest pie pan or biggest deep dish shell you can find.) Cover and seal with top pie crust making vent holes in at least 4 places. Bake for 45 minutes, or until top is golden brown.

Family Secret: This pie can be made and frozen. I double wrap mine in heavy foil. I make about 15 a year when the apple trees are loaded, and use them all winter long. Let frozen pie set out at room temperature for about 1 hour. Then bake according to recipe directions.

Roselyn B. Dulany
Clarksdale

APPLE CRUMB PIE

SERVES: 8   OVEN: 450°

4 large, tart apples   ½ cup sugar
½ cup sugar   ¾ cup all-purpose flour
1 teaspoon cinnamon   ⅓ cup margarine

Peel apples, cut in slices, and arrange in nine inch pie crust. Mix ½ cup sugar with cinnamon and sprinkle over apples. Sift remaining ½ cup of sugar with flour; cut in margarine until crumbly. Sprinkle over apples. Cover edges of pie crust with aluminum foil. Bake for 10 minutes; lower temperature to 350° and bake 40 additional minutes.

Mrs. Rick Parsons
Vance

MISS OLLIE'S CHERRY PIE

SERVES: 6   OVEN: 350°

1 cup sugar   1 tablespoon butter
¼ cup flour   ¼ teaspoon salt
½ cup juice   10 drops food coloring
1 can sour pitted cherries   1 double pie crust

Combine all ingredients except cherries. Bring to a boil, cook three minutes. Fold in cherries and add food color. Put into bottom of 8 inch pie crust. Top with remaining crust and flute. Cut 4 to 6 vents in top crust to allow steam to escape. Bake about 30 to 45 minutes.

Family Secret: My mother gave me this recipe that she has used for over fifty years.

Jo Ann White
Destin, Florida

FRESH PEACH COBBLER

SERVES: 4 TO 6   OVEN: 425°

4 cups sliced fresh peaches   ½ teaspoon salt
1 cup sugar   2 tablespoons butter
1 tablespoon lemon juice   2 layer pie crust recipe, cut
2 tablespoons flour   into strips
¼ teaspoon cinnamon

Sprinkle peaches in bowl with lemon juice. Mix sugar, flour, salt, and cinnamon together. Fold into peaches. Place ½ of peach mixture in 2 quart casserole dish and dot with butter. Cover with ½ of pastry strips. Place in oven lightly brown, (5 to 10 minutes). Add remainder of peach mixture; dot with butter; cover with other half of pastry strips and cook until brown. (25 minutes).

Faye Skewes
Clarksdale

OATMEAL PIE

SERVES: 6   OVEN: 375°

3 eggs, well beaten   ⅔ cup brown sugar
⅔ cup sugar   ⅔ cup oatmeal
⅔ cup coconut   ¼ cup butter
1 teaspoon vanilla   8 inch baked pie shell

Mix and bake 30 minutes.

James Wooddall

CUSTARD PIE

This recipe is 148 years old and has been passed through 6 generations. It has truly been tried and tested!

YIELD: 6 TO 8   OVEN: 375°

1 nine inch unbaked pie shell
½ cup sugar
⅓ cup flour
1 rounded teaspoon butter (original recipe said size of walnut)

1 teaspoon vanilla
2 to 3 eggs, beaten (depending on size of eggs)
2 cups milk
2 tablespoons sugar
Whole nutmeg, grate or grind the nutmeg

Prick crust with fork in 5 or 6 places. Mix sugar and flour. Spread on unbaked crust. Over this, crumble butter. Beat eggs in medium bowl. Add vanilla, milk, sugar, and mix. Pour into crust. Grate nutmeg on top. Bake for 25 - 30 minutes.

Eileen M. Casburn
Sumner

AUNT OPAL'S
OLD FASHIONED LEMON MERINGUE PIE

SERVES: 8 TO 10   OVEN: 350°

FILLING:
1½ cups sugar
½ cup cornstarch
1½ cups cold water

3 egg yolks
2 tablespoons butter
¼ cup lemon juice

Mix sugar, cornstarch, and water together. Cook over medium heat until mixture is clear. Mix ½ of mixture into 3 egg yolks. Mix well. Add remaining mixture. Cook 3 minutes. Add butter and blend well. Add lemon juice. Cool. Put in 10 inch baked pie shell.

MERINGUE:
3 egg whites
1 teaspoon water

½ teaspoon cream of tartar
3 tablespoons sugar

Combine egg whites, water, and cream of tartar. Beat until foamy. Add sugar. Beat until stiff. Smooth on top of lemon filling. Bake 10 minutes until lightly brown. Best served warm.

Jean Duff
Alligator

NANNY'S CARAMEL PIE

When Nanny went to the kitchen and pulled out that black iron skillet, we knew we were in for a treat!

SERVES: 6 TO 8   OVEN: 350°

½ cup sugar	½ cup of sugar
1 tablespoon flour	1 tablespoon very hot water
3 eggs	1 teaspoon vanilla
1¼ cups milk	1 tablespoon butter
Pinch of salt	1 baked 8 inch pie crust

Mix ½ cup of sugar with the flour. Beat 1 egg plus 2 egg yolks (save whites for making meringue) and add to sugar mixture. Add milk and salt, beating well with wire whisk. Set aside. Brown ½ cup sugar in a heavy pan. It is best to do this over medium heat allowing sugar to melt slowly. When completely dissolved, continue to cook until syrup is a golden color. Watch out! This will burn easily if overcooked. When sugar is browned add 1 tablespoon very hot water whisking constantly. Continue whisking as you slowly pour egg/milk mixture into browned sugar. Cook until thickened. Remove from heat and add vanilla and butter. Pour into baked pie crust and top with meringue made from remaining egg whites. Bake until meringue is lightly browned. Cool before serving.

Mrs. Hartley Kittle (Lynn)
Clarksdale

FUDGE PIE

SERVES: 8 TO 10   OVEN: 375°

1 cup butter or margarine, softened	½ cup flour
2 cups sugar	½ cup cocoa
4 eggs	1 cup nuts

Cream butter and sugar. Add eggs one at a time and beat after each one. Sift flour and cocoa into mixture. Add nuts. Pour into lightly greased 10 inch pie plate. Bake for 25 to 30 minutes or until crust forms on top. Serve with ice cream or whipped cream.

Maggie Tyner
Nelda Mooney
Clarksdale

BUTTERMILK COCONUT PIE

SERVES: 8   OVEN: 325°

1 stick butter
1¼ cups sugar
2 tablespoons flour
2 eggs
½ cup buttermilk

1½ cups coconut
1 teaspoon vanilla (I use 2
   teaspoons vanilla)
1 unbaked 9 inch pie shell

Melt butter. Set butter aside. Beat sugar, flour, and eggs well. Add buttermilk, butter, coconut, and vanilla. Pour in unbaked 9 inch pie shell and cook till crust is brown and the pie is firm, or 45 to 50 minutes.

Mrs. Oscar Bryant Wolfe
Duncan

HARTUNG'S SNACK BAR CREAM PIE

SERVES: 8

¾ cup sugar
⅔ cup non - fat dry milk
2 rounded tablespoons flour
3 rounded tablespoons
   cornstarch

2 egg yolks
2 cups water
1 teaspoon vanilla
1 tablespoon butter or
   margarine

Mix all of dry ingredients together (including cocoa for chocolate pie). Separate egg yolks. Put whites in a bowl for meringue. Add water very slowly to egg yolks and dry ingredient mixture, gradually mixing in all of dry ingredients and water. Cook over medium - low heat, stirring constantly, until thick (approximately 10 minutes). Stir vigorously through lumpy stage - mixture will be smooth when done. Remove from heat, add vanilla and butter. (Mix in coconut or pineapple for those pies.) Let cool. Put into baked pie shell. Put meringue on top. Bake at 350° until lightly browned.

VARIATIONS:
Banana Pie: 2 bananas sliced place on pie shell bottom before cream filling. Chocolate Pie: Add 3 tablespoons cocoa. Coconut Pie: Add ¼ cup flaked coconut to filling. Sprinkle coconut on top of meringue. Pineapple Pie: Add ¼ cup crushed pineapple (drained and blotted).

Family Secret: You can substitute 2 cups of milk for ⅔ cup dry milk and 2 cups water.

Jean Hartung Duff
Alligator

PAULETTE'S KAHLUA COFFEE PARFAIT PIE

SERVES: 8   OVEN: 375°

CRUST:

1 (7 ounce) package flaked coconut

2 tablespoons all purpose flour

4 ounces pecans, finely chopped

½ cup margarine, melted

Combine coconut, flour and pecans in large bowl. Add melted margarine and mix until all ingredients are well moistened. Press into 10 - inch metal pie pan with wooden spoon. Crust must be level with rim of pie pan to prevent burning when baking. Bake 10 minutes or until golden brown. Cool completely before adding filling.

FILLING:

1 quart coffee ice cream, softened

1 cup semi - sweet chocolate chips

½ pint heavy cream, whipped

Semi - sweet chocolate, grated

Fold chocolate chips into ice cream. Pack crust 2 to 3 inches deep with ice cream. Freeze. To serve, remove pie from freezer a few minutes before serving time. Place pie slices on individual plates, top with whipped cream and sprinkle with grated chocolate. Pour 1 ounce of Kahlua on each slice just before serving.

George Falls
Paulette's Restaurant
Memphis, Tennessee

PECAN COCONUT PIE

SERVES: 8   OVEN: 350°

1 cup sugar

1 cup dark corn syrup

½ teaspoon salt

⅓ cup melted butter

1½ tablespoons corn meal

1 teaspoon vanilla

3 eggs

¾ cup shredded coconut

1 cup pecans, whole or chopped

Mix syrup, sugar, salt, butter, vanilla, and corn meal. Add slightly beaten eggs. Pour into unbaked 9 inch pie shell. Sprinkle coconut over fillings, then pecans. Bake for 45 minutes.

Roberta DeFord
Clarksdale

PECAN PIE

SERVES: 8   OVEN: 400°

1 unbaked 9 - inch pie shell	1 teaspoon vanilla
3 eggs beaten	1 cup sugar
1 cup dark corn syrup	2 tablespoons melted butter
⅛ teaspoon salt	1 cup chopped pecans

Mix all ingredients together in bowl with spoon and pour into 1 unbaked pie shell and bake at 400° for first 10 minutes, then turn temperature down to 350° and cook for another 40 minutes.

Family Secret: To keep outside edge of crust on pie from turning too dark while baking, cut aluminum foil strips and cover pie crust edge.

Meg Agostinelli
Lyon

RASPBERRY PIE

SERVES: 8   OVEN: 300°

CRUST:

1⅓ cups crushed graham crackers	3 tablespoons powdered sugar
¼ cup margarine, melted	

Combine graham crackers, margarine, and sugar; and mix well. Pat into a 9 inch pie plate.

FILLING:

8 ounces cream cheese, softened	1 teaspoon vanilla
2 eggs	½ cup sugar

Combine next 4 ingredients and pour into pie shell. Bake for 15 to 18 minutes. Cool.

TOPPING:

10 ounces frozen raspberries, thawed	3 tablespoons sugar
	2 tablespoons cornstarch

Purée and strain raspberries to remove seeds. Put into saucepan, add sugar and cornstarch. Cook over medium heat to thicken. Cool. Spread on pie. Top with whipped cream.

Leeba McElroy
Clarksdale

CHESS PIE

SERVES: 4 TO 6   OVEN: 350°

1 unbaked pie shell
½ cup margarine, melted
3 eggs
1½ cups sugar

2 tablespoons corn meal
1½ teaspoons vinegar
1 teaspoon vanilla

Mix above well. Bake in an uncooked pie shell for 45 minutes.

Mrs. Lee Graves
Clarksdale

KEY LIME PIE

SERVES: 6 TO 8

4 egg yolks
1 (14 ounce) can sweetened
   condensed milk
3 ounces key lime juice

8-inch graham cracker crust
1 cup whipping cream,
   whipped

Combine yolks, milk and mix well. Add lime juice slowly. Pour into crust. Top with whipped cream.

Georgia Haaga
Clarksdale

MAMA'S PIE CRUST

My parent's plate lunches and pies drew the business community for lunch in downtown Pine Bluff, Arkansas for years. Mama's original recipes were closely guarded secrets until after their retirement.

YIELD: 4 8-INCH CRUSTS   OVEN: 400°

2 cups all purpose flour
1 teaspoon salt
¾ cup shortening (4 heaping
   tablespoons)

⅓ cup cold water

Add salt to flour in large bowl. Add shortening. Mix well with pastry blender. Add water, work together with hands until smooth. Can be divided into 4 parts to make four small pie crusts, 2 double crust pies or three large pie crusts. Crusts can be frozen in patties, thawed and rolled out, or put into pie pans and then frozen. Unfilled crusts for cream pies are baked, 10 to 12 minutes.

Jean Hartung Duff
Alligator

QUICK APRICOT PASTRIES

SERVES: 24 OVEN: 425°

1 package refrigerator crescent rolls (8 roll size)
½ cup apricot jam or favorite
  flavor

1 cup sour cream
1 beaten egg
1 tablespoon sugar

Unroll crescent rolls. Pat into bottom of buttered (or sprayed with cooking spray) 13 x 9 inch glass baking dish. Spread with jam. Bake for 15 minutes. Remove from oven. Reduce heat to 325°. Combine remaining ingredients. Pour evenly over rolls, bake 5 to 6 minutes more. Cut in small squares. Serve warm. Great for brunch.

Verne Kittell

BEST COOKIES YOU EVER ATE

YIELD: 3 TO 4 DOZEN OVEN: 350°

1 cup vegetable shortening
2 eggs
2 cups sugar
3 tablespoons molasses
2 teaspoons cinnamon
2 cups plain flour

1½ teaspoons salt
2 teaspoons baking soda
⅔ cup chopped pecans
1½ cups raisins
2 cups oatmeal

Combine shortening, eggs, sugar, molasses and cinnamon in mixer. Beat until smooth. Sift together flour, baking soda, and salt. Add to first mixture. Beat until well combined. Add oatmeal, pecans and raisins. Drop by heaping teaspoon on greased cookie sheet. Bake for 8 minutes.

Mrs. Sylvia S. Murphey
Sumner

KOURABREDES (BUTTER COOKIES)

This is a traditional Greek dessert for New Year's Day.

YIELD: 3 TO 4 DOZEN OVEN: 350°

1 pound whipped sweet
  unsalted butter
½ cup sugar
2 egg yolks
1 small jigger bourbon

2 teaspoons vanilla
2 pounds plain flour
1 teaspoon baking powder
1 pound confectioner's sugar

CONTINUED, KOURABREDES (BUTTER COOKIES)

Cream butter with sugar. Add egg yolks and beat until light. Add bourbon and vanilla. Sift flour and baking powder. Add to creamed mixture. Knead well by hand to form a stiff dough. If dough requires more liquid, add a few drops of bourbon. If it is too soft, add a little flour. Mix well and shape into small balls, or roll to ¼ inch thickness and cut to any desired shape with cookie cutters. For easier shaping, let dough be cooled; line the butter cookies on a greased cookie sheet and bake in oven for about 20 minutes. When cool, remove to a large platter in layers. Dust each layer generously with confectioner's sugar. Cookies stay fresh for 2 to 3 weeks.

Mary Beth Peters
Clarksdale

FRUIT CAKE COOKIES

YIELD: 3 DOZEN   OVEN: 325°

FRUIT MIXTURE:

½ pound red candied cherries	½ pound dates
½ pound green candied cherries	4 cups pecans
½ pound red candied pineapples	

Chop fruit and nuts. Pour 7 tablespoons whiskey over fruit and let it stand overnight.

DOUGH MIXTURE:

1½ sticks margarine, softened	1 teaspoon each cinnamon and allspice
½ cup brown sugar	1 teaspoon baking powder
2 eggs, beaten	¼ teaspoon salt
1 teaspoon soda, dissolved in 1 tablespoon water	2 cups flour

Cream margarine and sugar. Add eggs and soda, dissolved in water. Stir together spices, baking powder, salt, and flour. Add to creamed mixture. Pour over fruit mixture which has been prepared in advance. Mix well. Drop by teaspoon on greased cookie sheet. Bake 12 minutes.

Family Secret: Not hard, but time consuming. However, they are delicious and make wonderful Christmas gifts for friends and neighbors.

Mary Eva Presley
Clarksdale

CHOCOLATE STAR PEANUT BUTTER COOKIES

YIELD: 5 DOZEN   OVEN: 375°

1½ cups all-purpose flour
1 teaspoon baking soda
⅛ teaspoon salt
½ cup (1 stick) margarine, softened
½ cup creamy peanut butter
1 cup granulated sugar (divided)

½ cup firmly packed brown sugar
1 egg
1 teaspoon vanilla extract
Chocolate candy stars or jellies

In small bowl stir together flour, baking soda, and salt. In large bowl of electric mixer at medium speed, beat margarine and peanut butter until well blended. Beat in ½ cup granulated sugar and brown sugar until blended. Beat in egg and vanilla. Reduce speed to low; gradually beat in flour mixture until well mixed. Shape dough into 1 inch balls; roll in remaining granulated sugar. Place on ungreased cookie sheets 2 inches apart. Bake for 10 minutes or until lightly browned. Remove from oven and quickly press a chocolate star firmly into top of each cookie (cookies will crack around the edges). Remove from cookie sheets. Cool.

Meg Agostinelli
Lyon

DATE BARS

SERVES: 16   OVEN: 325°

2 eggs
1 cup confectioner's sugar
1 tablespoon shortening, melted
¼ cup sifted flour

½ teaspoon baking powder
¼ teaspoon salt
1 cup chopped dates
¾ cup pecans, chopped
1 teaspoon vanilla

Beat eggs until light. Add sugar and shortening. Blend well. Sift dry ingredients together, add to first mixture. Add dates, nuts, and vanilla. Blend well and pour into greased 8 x 8 inch pan. Bake 25 minutes.

Rita Moser
Clarksdale

ROSETTES

YIELD: 2 TO 3 DOZEN

2 cups flour
1 cup evaporated milk
1 cup water
2 tablespoons sugar

1 teaspoon salt
1 tablespoon orange extract
2 eggs, unbeaten

Mix in order all ingredients until smooth. Use tempered pastry iron, which usually comes in 2 designs. This can be purchased at department stores and directions for tempering irons are on the box. Pour 1 to 1½ inches vegetable oil into heavy skillet. Heat to very hot but not smoking. Dip pastry iron into batter (do not cover top of iron) and dip into deep skillet of hot oil. Use long fork to loosen pastry from iron. Brown lightly on each side (few seconds). Place each Rosette on cookies sheet which has been lined with paper towels to absorb the oil. When cool, put in a tightly covered container for storage. When you are ready to or serve, top each Rosette with honey and crushed pecans. Then sprinkle with cinnamon.

Jean Paulos Ellington
Memphis, Tennessee

AUSTRIAN JAM COOKIES

YIELD: 2 DOZEN   OVEN: 300°

½ cup softened butter
½ cup sugar
1 teaspoon vanilla
1 separated egg

1¼ cups sifted all purpose
    flour
⅔ cup chopped almonds
Raspberry jam

Beat butter, sugar, vanilla and egg yolk in a medium-sized bowl until fluffy. Stir in flour; gather dough into a ball; chill several hours. Roll level teaspoon of dough into balls. Dip into slightly beaten egg white; roll in almonds. Place on ungreased cookie sheet one inch apart. Press an indentation with finger in each; fill with jam. Bake in a slow oven for twenty minutes or until lightly golden. Cool on wire racks.

Sue P. Bell
Clarksdale

CHESS SQUARES

YIELD: 24   OVEN 350°

1 box chocolate or yellow
  butter cake mix
1 egg
½ cup margarine or butter,
  softened

3 eggs
1 package (8 ounce) cream
  cheese, softened
1 teaspoon vanilla
1 pound powdered sugar

Mix first three ingredients and spread in greased 9 x 13 inch pan. Beat eggs and add remaining ingredients. Pour over first layer. Bake for 30 to 40 minutes. Cool and cut into squares.

Peggy Beckham
Clarksdale

CHESS NOELS

YIELD: 5 TO 6 DOZEN   OVEN: 350°

¾ cup margarine, softened
1½ cups sifted flour
3 tablespoons granulated
  sugar
2¼ cups (1 pound) dark
  brown sugar, packed

3 egg yolks, beaten
1 cup coarsely chopped
  pecans
½ teaspoon vanilla
3 egg whites, beaten stiffly
2 cups powdered sugar

Cream margarine. Add flour and granulated sugar slowly. Mix well. Spread on bottom of cookie sheet (15½ x 10½ inches x 1 inch). Bake for 10 to 15 minutes. Mix brown sugar with beaten egg yolks thoroughly. Add pecans and vanilla. Fold in stiffly beaten egg whites. Spread evenly over baked layer, being sure to cover corners. Return to oven for 15 to 20 minutes. Do not over bake. Dust with sifted powdered sugar. Cool. Cut into bars.

Emily Cooper
Clarksdale

LATOUGI - ITALIAN COOKIES

YIELD: 10 TO 12 DOZEN

6 cups flour	⅓ stick or 2½ tablespoons
6 eggs	butter, melted
⅔ cup sugar	Oil for frying
4 teaspoons vanilla	Confectioner's sugar

Sift flour. Mix next 4 ingredients together. Pour into sifted flour. Make dough to consistency to roll out thin enough to cut with pastry cutter. (It's important to roll as thin as possible). Cut into squares approximately 3 x 3 inches. Cut four slits in center of each square. Turn ends to second slit and pull through gently. Have oil deep enough in frying pan so that dough will float when put in. Heat oil to frying temperature. Cook until light brown (1 to 1½ minutes). Take out, drain, and sprinkle with confectioner's sugar if desired.

Regina Youngblood
Clarksdale

OATMEAL COOKIES

YIELD: 3 TO 4 DOZEN   OVEN: 350°

1 cup brown sugar	1½ cups flour
1 cup sugar	1 teaspoon baking soda
1 cup butter or margarine,	1 teaspoon salt
softened	3 cups oatmeal
2 eggs	½ cup chopped pecans
1 teaspoon vanilla	

Soften butter, mix with sugars, beat in eggs with mixer. Add vanilla. Sift dry ingredients together, then add to mixture. Add oatmeal and chopped nuts, stirring until mixed well. Drop by teaspoons on cookie sheet. Bake 8 to 12 minutes or until VERY LIGHTLY BROWNED.

Jean Duff, Nancy Olson, Kathy Davis
Clarksdale

PECAN CHEWY

YIELD: 2 DOZEN   OVEN: 325°

4 eggs, slightly beaten   1½ cups all purpose flour
½ stick butter or margarine   1½ teaspoons baking powder
1 box (1 pound) brown sugar   2 cups chopped pecans

Combine in saucepan over low heat eggs, butter, and sugar. Mix
flour, baking powder, and pecans. Add to egg mixture and stir until
blended. Spread into greased 13 x 9 inch pan. Bake 40 minutes. Cut
into squares after cooling to serve.

Family Secret: Good as a light dessert, or snack or for a coffee or tea.

Shirley Easley
Clarksdale

FAT LADIES

SERVES: 25 TO 30   OVEN: 350°

1 roll chocolate chip cookie   35 caramels
   dough   10 ounces chocolate chips
½ cup half and half   1 cup pecans

Preheat oven. In 9 x 12 inch pan, put cookies ¼ inch deep. Flatten.
Cook for 12 to 14 minutes. Melt caramels with half and half in
microwave. Put chocolate chips over cookie layer. Cook until
chocolate is melted about 5 minutes or more. Spread caramel mixture
evenly. Sprinkle pecans on top. Cool. Cut into bars.

Nelda Mooney
Friars Point

SCOTCH SHORT BREAD

YIELD: 12 TO 15   OVEN: 325°

1 cup butter (no substitute)   2 cups unsifted flour
   at room temperature   2 tablespoons either corn-
½ cup granulated sugar   starch or rice flour

CONTINUED, SCOTCH SHORT BREAD

Cream butter thoroughly, add sugar gradually, creaming until smooth. Add flour to which cornstarch or rice flour has been added. Work with hands or wooden spoon. Use only as much flour as needed to make a stiff dough (I use all the flour). Cover and chill overnight for finer texture or use immediately. Flatten dough on lightly floured surface to ¼ inch thickness. This may be cut into desired shape and size or flattened in pie pan and cut in pie-shaped sections. Place in ungreased pan. Prick with fork, bake for 30 minutes or until lightly browned. Melts in your mouth or keeps well in cookie jar.

Margaret S. Craig
Friars Point

CREOLE LACE COOKIES

YIELD: 2 TO 3 DOZEN   OVEN: 325°

1 cup quick oatmeal	1 cup sugar
3 tablespoons flour, unsifted	1 stick butter (no substitute)
½ teaspoon baking powder	1 tablespoon vanilla
1 teaspoon salt	1 egg, beaten

Mix dry ingredients. Cut in butter; add vanilla and egg. Mix well and refrigerate overnight. Drop marble sized pieces of dough on cookie sheet lined with foil, about 3 inches apart as they spread during cooking. Bake about 11 minutes. Do not let them get too dark. Cool just enough to peel cookies off foil, then cool thoroughly and store in an air-tight container.

Joyce Paslay
Clarksdale

REFRIGERATOR COOKIES

YIELD: 3 TO 4 DOZEN   OVEN: 375°

1 tablespoon milk	2 eggs, beaten
2 sticks margarine (softened)	2 teaspoons vanilla
2 cups sugar (1 white, 1 brown)	3 cups flour (2 cups self-rising, 1 cup plain)
½ teaspoon baking soda	1½ cups chopped pecans

Mix all ingredients in order given. Put on wax paper. Roll up and chill or freeze. Slice and bake as needed. (Roll about the size of a Silver Dollar. Slice in ½ inch to ¾ inch slices.) Bake approximately 15 minutes or until browned. Do not double.

Evelyn W. Butler
Alligator

DELICIOUS HOLIDAY COOKIES

YIELD: 2 TO 3 DOZEN   OVEN: 300°

1 cup margarine, softened
4 tablespoons powdered
  sugar
2 teaspoons of vanilla

2 cups cake flour
2 cups finely chopped pecans
Powdered sugar

Beat margarine until soft. Add sugar and blend until creamy. Add vanilla and flour. Stir in pecans. Roll dough into small balls. Flatten slightly and place on cookies sheet. Bake for 35 to 40 minutes until golden. Roll in powdered sugar while still hot and again when cooled. Store in air-tight container.

Cathy Middleton
Clarksdale

AUNT BESSIE'S SUGAR COOKIES

YIELD: 4 OR 5 DOZEN   OVEN: 325°

2 sticks butter, softened
1 cup sugar
1 beaten egg
2 cups flour

½ teaspoon cream of tartar
½ teaspoon baking soda
1 teaspoon vanilla

Cream butter and sugar. Add egg. Add flour mixed with soda and cream of tartar. Add vanilla. Make into a roll, wrap in wax paper, and chill overnight. Take out and slice. Put on two lightly greased cookie sheets. Cook approximately 10 to 15 minutes depending on oven.

Joyce Paslay
Clarksdale

CHOCOLATE DECORATION ICING

YIELD: ¾ CUP

1 ounce unsweetened
  chocolate
1 teaspoon butter or
  margarine

1 cup sifted powdered sugar
1 tablespoon hot water

Melt chocolate and butter in top of double boiler. Remove from heat. Stir in sugar and water, a teaspoon at a time, until desired consistency. To be used in a decorator's tube.

Margie Cooper
Clarksdale

ROBERT E. LEE COOKIES

YIELD: ABOUT 5 DOZEN   OVEN: 350°

1½ cups (3 sticks) margarine,   4 cups sifted plain flour
   melted   4 teaspoons soda
½ cup molasses   2 teaspoons cinnamon
2 cups sugar   1 teaspoon ginger
2 eggs   1 teaspoon cloves

Combine margarine, molasses, sugar and eggs. With electric mixer beat well. Sift dry ingredients and add to first mixture. Refrigerate dough for several hours. Make into small balls and roll in granulated sugar. Bake on ungreased cookie sheet until firm and brown, about 8 to 10 minutes.

Louise Nix
Clarksdale

TEA CAKES

Grandmother Butler always kept tea cake dough in the refrigerator. Living on a farm, we never knew who would show up as a guest for dinner.

YIELD: APPROXIMATELY 8 DOZEN   OVEN: 350°

2 cups sugar   1 cup shortening
½ cup buttermilk   1 teaspoon salt
3 eggs   1 teaspoon vanilla flavoring
1 teaspoon soda   6 cups flour

Mix all ingredients before adding flour. Use enough flour to make stiff dough, adding one cup at at time until you have added 5 cups. After that, add in increments of ¼ cup until you have a stiff dough. Roll out thin, approximately ⅛ inch thickness, and cut large cookies. Bake for approximately 15 to 20 minutes or until brown on top.

Barbara Butler Graves
Clarksdale

DECORATING ICING

YIELD: ¾ CUP

2 cups powdered sugar   1 tablespoon water

Mix sugar and water. Add more water 1 teaspoon at at time until icing is of consistency that can be used easily in a decorator's tube and still hold its shape.

Margie Cooper
Clarksdale

SCRUMPTIOUS APRICOT SOUFFLÉ

SERVES: 8 TO 10   OVEN: 375°

½ pound dried apricots
2½ cups water
1 cup superfine sugar
3 tablespoons lemon juice

7 large egg whites
Pinch of salt
Confectioner's sugar

Put the apricots and 1½ cups of water in a 2 - quart saucepan, and let stand for 2 hours. Add the remaining cup of water, bring the mixture to a boil over moderate heat, cover and cook for 20 minutes. Use the metal blade of a food processor to process the mixture until smooth, about 45 seconds, stopping once to scrape down the bowl. Strain the purée through a sieve into a 3 - quart mixing bowl. Stir in ¾ cup of sugar and 2 tablespoons lemon juice. Let the mixture cool and then refrigerate it, covered, for at least 1 hour. Butter and sugar freezer-to-oven soufflé molds, 8 of the 1-cup size or 10 to 12 smaller ones. Refrigerate the molds for about ½ hour. With a wire whisk or an electric mixer, beat the egg whites with a pinch of salt until soft peaks form. Gradually beat in the remaining ¼ cup sugar and then 1 tablespoon lemon juice. Continue to beat the mixture until it forms stiff and shiny peaks. Stir 1 cup of the egg whites into the apricot purée. Then fold the mixture back into the egg whites with a large rubber spatula. Pour into the prepared molds, mounding the mixture about 1 inch above the rim. Shape into a cone with a small metal spatula. Make a groove with your finger about a quarter of the way in from the edge of the mold. Bring the mixture up and let it fall off the end of your finger to form a topknot. Smooth the edge with a small knife and wipe off the rim of the mold. The filled molds may be refrigerated for up to an hour. Put the soufflés in a shallow baking pan and add enough hot water to reach ⅓ of the way up the sides of the molds. Bake for 30 minutes in the preheated oven. Remove the soufflés from the pan of water and sift confectioner's sugar over the tops. With a tablespoon remove the tops of the soufflés, fill the cavities with 2 to 3 tablespoons of custard. Replace lids and serve immediately.

CONTINUED, SCRUMPTIOUS APRICOT SOUFFLÉ

CUSTARD:

4 medium egg yolks	2 cups milk, scalded
¼ cup sugar	2 teaspoons orange liqueur
⅛ teaspoon salt	

Blend sugar, salt and slightly beaten egg yolks. Pour ½ cup of milk into egg mixture; blend. Pour all of egg-milk mixture into top of double boiler with rest of milk. Cook, stirring constantly, over simmering water until it is thick enough to coat a spoon. Remove from heat and add liqueur. Strain to remove lumps and chill.

Family Secret: Big Bonus: Soufflés can be frozen and put directly into 350° oven for 35 to 40 minutes.

Jennie Neblett
Clarksdale

BEST BANANA PUDDING

SERVES: 8

¾ cup sugar	
2 tablespoons flour	2 egg yolks, lightly beaten
2 tablespoons cornstarch	1 teaspoon vanilla flavoring
2 cups milk (May substitute	1 tablespoon butter
⅔ cup non-fat dry milk	2 bananas, sliced
plus 2 cups water instead	Vanilla wafers
of milk)	

Mix first three ingredients in saucepan. Put ½ cup of dry ingredients in another bowl and add egg yolks and milk. Add milk very slowly and carefully while mixing. Add liquid mixture to remaining dry mix in saucepan. Cook over medium low heat until thick, approximately 10 minutes, stirring constantly.Remove from heat and add vanilla and butter. Allow butter to melt. Mix well. Cover the bottom of a 9 x 9 inch dish with vanilla wafers, then add banana. Pour pudding into dish. Put vanilla wafers around side of dish. Crumble vanilla wafers on top. EAT WHILE WARM!

Jean Hartung Duff
Alligator

ALMOND BISQUE

SERVES: 9

¾ cup graham cracker crumbs
22 large marshmallows
½ cup milk

2 teaspoons almond extract
½ pint whipping cream
½ cup graham cracker crumbs

Spread graham cracker crumbs on bottom of buttered 8-inch square pan. Pour milk over marshmallows in a double boiler. Cook on medium heat until marshmallows are melted, being careful not to get mixture too hot. When marshmallows are melted, cool pan in ice water. Add almond extract. Whip cream and fold into marshmallow mixture. Spread mixture over graham cracker crumbs and sprinkle remaining crumbs on top. Freeze. May be doubled or tripled.

Toni Malvezzi Hardin
Duncan

FOUR-LAYER DESSERT

SERVES: 12 TO 15   OVEN: 350°

1 cup all-purpose flour
½ cup margarine, softened
1½ cups chopped pecans
   (divided)
2 cups frozen whipped non-
   dairy topping (divided)
1 (8 ounce) package cream
   cheese, softened

1 cup powdered sugar
1 (6¾ ounce) package instant
   vanilla pudding
1 (6¾ ounce) package instant
   chocolate pudding
3 cups cold milk

Cream flour and margarine together. Add 1 cup nuts. Press into 9 x 12 inch pan. Bake 20 minutes. Cool completely. Cream 1 cup frozen whipped topping, cream cheese, and sugar. Spread over first layer. Combine both pudding mixes and milk in mixing bowl. Mix until thick; spread over second layer. Cover third layer with remaining frozen whipped topping and sprinkle with ½ cup chopped pecans. Much better if allowed to stand, covered, in refrigerator overnight.

Susan Connell, Rita Moser, Alberta Crawford
Clarksdale

LOG CABIN DESSERT

SERVES: 6 TO 8

¾ cup butter, softened
4 egg yolks
2 cups powdered sugar
3 tablespoons strong coffee
1 teaspoon vanilla

1 dozen lady fingers,
  separated
Whipped cream
Maraschino cherries

Cream butter, egg yolks, and sugar. Add coffee and vanilla. Arrange lady finger halves in a triangle on individual dessert plates. Put creamed mixture in center and top with whipped cream and a cherry. This may also be served by lining a large silver or glass bowl with the lady fingers and filling the center with cream.

Baby Doll Peacock Walker (Mrs. Ben, Jr.)
Tribbett

NEGRESSE EN CHEMISE

SERVES: 10

1 ounce unsweetened block
  chocolate
11 ounces semi-sweet block
  chocolate
4 fluid ounces strong black
  coffee
¼ cup rum or brandy or to
  taste

3 ounces or 6 tablespoons of
  unsalted butter, softened
4 ounces praline, crushed
  fine, or substitute crushed
  almond or cashew brittle
¾ pint double cream, divided

Gently melt chocolate with coffee and brandy. Beat butter and praline, pour in liquid chocolate (not too hot), mix well and fold in half the cream (whipped but not too firm). Pour into mold and chill 3 to 4 hours. Use 1 pint bombe mold well oiled. Turn out and decorate with remaining cream. Do not freeze.

Edwin Mullens
Lyon

CRÈME BRULÉE

SERVES: 12   OVEN: 350°

This recipe is from the Inn For All Seasons located between Burford and Sherborne in England.

2 pints double cream
8 egg yolks
Some vanilla essence (about 2
   teaspoons vanilla extract)

4 tablespoons caster sugar
   (fine granulated sugar)
Demerara sugar for topping
   (coarse brown sugar)

Heat cream in heavy pan or double boiler until nearly boiling. Lightly whisk egg yolks, sugar, and vanilla in large bowl. Gradually whisk in cream. Put 12 crème brulée pots on baking sheet with at least 1 inch sides. Surround with water half way of sides of pots. Fill the pots with the mixture and place in oven for approximately 30 minutes on Gas no. 5. When cool, put a thin layer of demerara sugar on top of the mixture and grill (broil) until caramelized.

Wert Cooper
Clarksdale

DEATH BY CHOCOLATE

SERVES: 18   OVEN: 350°

1 box chocolate cake mix
1 cup Kahlua coffee liqueur
4 boxes chocolate mousse
   mix

2 (12-ounce) tubs whipped
   topping
6 chocolate-toffee candy bars
   (broken into small pieces)

Bake cake according to package directions for 9 x 12 inch cake. Prick top of baked cake with fork: pour Kahlua over the cake. Let this soak in (it can be left this way overnight). Make the chocolate mousse according to package directions. To assemble cake: Crumble up half of the baked cake and place it on bottom of large glass bowl. Layer half of mousse; then half of whipped topping; and half of the candy bar pieces. Repeat layers.

Family Secret: This is great for a party or barbecue! Put in a pretty, clear glass dish so that you can see the different layers.

Carolyn Stringer
Clarksdale

SPECIAL CHARLOTTE FOR SPECIAL GUESTS

SERVES: 8

2 tablespoons plain gelatin
1 cup cold water, divided
4 egg yolks, well beaten
1 cup sugar
Pinch of salt

1 quart whipping cream, whipped
2 tablespoons brandy, rum or bourbon (optional)
2 dozen ladyfingers

Dissolve gelatin in ½ cup cold water. Let stand 15 minutes. Add rest of water. Cook in top of double boiler 10 minutes. Combine beaten egg yolks, sugar and salt. Gradually add to gelatin, mixing well. Cook until custard coats the spoon. Set aside to cool, but not harden. When cool, fold in whipped cream and alcohol (optional). Line 2 quart crystal dish or other 2 quart mold with ladyfingers and spoon custard mixture in. Refrigerate overnight. Unmold and/or garnish with strawberries and holly or mint.

Family Secret: Should be prepared only 1 day ahead.

Jane Longino
Clarksdale

BOILED CUSTARD

SERVES: 2 TO 3

2 well beaten eggs
2 cups sweet milk

¼ cup sugar
1 teaspoon vanilla

Blend first three ingredients together and cook slowly. Stir constantly while cooking. When spoon is nearly coated, remove from heat and add one teaspoon of vanilla flavoring. Pour into custard cups and serve warm or cold.

Rita Moser
Clarksdale

LEMON LOAF WITH RASPBERRY SAUCE

SERVES: 20 TO 25

3 cups sugar
3 envelopes plain gelatin
½ teaspoon salt
3 cups water
9 eggs, separated-save 4
  whites

1 tablespoon freshly grated
  lemon peel (or ½
  tablespoon dried)
¾ cup lemon juice
1 cup sugar, divided
4 cups whipped cream

Grease a 15½ x 4 x 4 inch loaf pan with butter and line bottom only with wax paper. In saucepan combine sugar with gelatin and salt. Stir in water. Beat egg yolks (reserve 4 whites in separate bowl); add to gelatin mixture. Cook over medium heat stirring constantly until it becomes a thin custard just coating a silver spoon. Remove from heat. If mixture is not smooth, beat with rotary beater. Stir in lemon peel and juice. Cool mixture until thickened but not set. Beat egg whites and gradually add ½ cup sugar. Beat until stiff peaks form. Beat whipping cream adding ½ cup sugar and continue beating until stiff peaks form. Fold whites into whipping cream and then into lemon mixture. Turn into mold. Refrigerate until set - 4 to 5 hours or overnight. Unmold and garnish with fresh mint leaves and whole raspberries.

RASPBERRY SAUCE:
1 pound fresh or frozen
  raspberries
½ cup water
1 cup sugar

1 tablespoon lemon juice
2 to 3 tablespoons Grand
  Marnier

Boil raspberries with water, sugar, and lemon juice until berries tear to pieces. Stir frequently. You may need a little more water but be careful not to add so much that the clear red color is destroyed. Strain to remove seeds. Add Grand Marnier to taste. Chill. Pour around base of unmolded lemon loaf or pass.

Leeba McElroy
Clarksdale

BAKED ALASKA

SERVES: 8   OVEN: 450°

9-inch baked pie shell in tin   1 (12 ounce) package semi-
  pie pan   sweet chocolate chips
2 pints peppermint ice   1⅓ cups evaporated milk
  cream, divided and   3 egg whites
  softened   6 tablespoons sugar

Bake pie shell in tin pan and allow to cool. Spread 1 pint ice cream
in pie shell and allow to harden in freezer. Make fudge sauce by
melting chocolate in double boiler or microwave and adding milk.
Cover ice cream with 1 cup fudge sauce. Place in freezer and when
sauce is hard, add second pint of ice cream and freeze. Beat egg
whites to which sugar has been added and put on top of pie being
very careful to seal edges. At time of serving, place in oven for 3
minutes. Serve with remainder of hot fudge sauce.

Donna Merkel
Clarksdale

SUGAR PLUM PUDDING

SERVES: 12   OVEN: 350°

PUDDING:
2 cups flour   1 cup buttermilk
1½ cups sugar   3 eggs
1¼ teaspoons soda   ¾ cup vegetable oil
1 teaspoon cinnamon   1 cup cooked, chopped
1 teaspoon allspice   prunes

Sift dry ingredients into large mixing bowl. Add other ingredients
and mix until blended. Bake for 40 minutes in a greased and floured
bundt pan. Serve hot with a generous spoonful of sauce.

SAUCE:
1 cup sugar   ½ cup buttermilk
½ cup margarine   1 teaspoon vanilla

Mix all ingredients in saucepan. Bring to boil. Serve warm or at
room temperature over warm plum pudding.

Sherry Donald
Clarksdale

BREAD PUDDING WITH WHISKEY SAUCE

SERVES: 10   OVEN: 350°

½ cup butter or margarine,   1 cup water
  softened   1 teaspoon vanilla extract
1½ cups sugar   1 pinch of salt
3 eggs   2 small loaves French Bread
1 (13 ounce) can evaporated   or 2 cups crumbs
  milk

Using electric mixer, cream butter and sugar; add eggs one at a time. Add milk, water, vanilla, and salt. This will look curdled. Pour ½ of mixture into an 8 x 8 inch baking dish. Break bread into small pieces and put in liquid in baking dish. When full of bread pieces, top with remaining liquid, making sure all bread is saturated. Bake for 45 minutes. Serve with whiskey sauce.

WHISKEY SAUCE:

YIELD: 1½ CUPS

1½ cups sugar   2 tablespoons margarine
1 (5.33 ounce) can evaporated   1 egg, beaten
  milk   2 tablespoons whiskey

Combine all ingredients except whiskey in top of double boiler. Place over boiling water and cook, stirring well, until thick. Keep warm until serving time or make ahead and refrigerate. Do not add whiskey until just before serving.

Mrs. Ted Roberts (Sheila)
Clarksdale

DESSERT PIZZA

SERVES: 8 TO 12   OVEN: 375°

½ cup butter or margarine,   ½ cup sour cream
  softened   ¼ cup lemon juice
¼ cup brown sugar   1 teaspoon vanilla
1 cup flour   2 to 3 pints any combination
¼ cup oats   of fresh fruit
¼ cup chopped nuts   Whipped cream for garnish
1 (14 ounce) can sweetened
  condensed milk

DESSERTS

CONTINUED, DESSERT PIZZA

Combine butter or margarine, brown sugar, flour, oats and nuts in mixing bowl. Spread on 12 inch pizza pan to form crust. Bake for 10 to 12 minutes. Combine sweetened condensed milk, sour cream, lemon juice, and vanilla in mixing bowl. Chill this combination until crust is baked and cooled. Remove creamy mixture from refrigerator and spread on crust. In a circular fashion top with sliced strawberries, peaches, blueberries, kiwi, pineapple, bananas, or whatever fruit suits your fancy. Optional garnish whipped cream and chopped nuts.

Family Secret: Plain or vanilla low-fat yogurt may be substituted for sour cream. This pizza is eye-catching, served either as a dessert or as a party food.

Sara Lynn Massey
Marks

MA BREWERS CUBAN FLAN

SERVES: 8   OVEN: 325°

6 eggs
1½ cups sugar
1 (11 ounce) can evaporated
  milk
1 (5 ounce) can evaporated
  milk

Dash of salt
1 teaspoon vanilla
1½ - 2 cups sugar
  (Depending on amount of
  syrup wanted)

Mix sugar and eggs together gently, without beating (beating can ruin recipe). Slowly add milk, again mixing gently with spoon. Add salt and vanilla. Meanwhile, melt down 1½ cups sugar in iron skillet (no butter or water necessary). Melt slowly until smooth and syrupy. Don't Panic! Pour syrup into a 1½ quart flan mold. Swirl syrup around to coat bottom well. Pour egg mixture into flan molds. Cover with aluminum foil (tightly, so no air gets in because this could also ruin your recipe). Place mold on a cookie sheet filled with water. Bake 1½ hours.

Family Secret: May be prepared the day before. Refrigerate until ready to serve. Invert on serving plate. You may decorate the center with flowers or holly around Christmas time.

Jennie Lowrence Neblett
Clarksdale

BLUEBERRY MERINGUES

YIELD: 8 TO 10   OVEN: 250°

2 egg whites   ⅛ teaspoon salt
½ teaspoon cream of tartar   ¼ teaspoon vanilla
½ cup sugar   1 cup blueberries

Beat egg whites and cream of tartar until stiff. Slowly add sugar, salt, and vanilla and continue beating until glossy and it forms stiff peaks. Fold in blueberries. Drop by tablespoons 2 inches apart on cookie sheet lined with parchment paper. Bake for 45 minutes. Cool 5 minutes and store in air-tight container.

Family Secret: Best if eaten day of preparation. Do not make on rainy day.

Eileen Casburn
Sumner

QUICK APPLE CRISP

SERVES: 6   OVEN: 350°

1 (20 ounce) can sliced apples   ¼ cup all-purpose flour
4 tablespoons butter   ¼ teaspoon salt
1 cup quick oats   ½ teaspoon cinnamon
½ cup brown sugar

Put sliced apples in an 8-inch square baking dish. In a medium bowl combine the oats, brown sugar, flour, salt and cinnamon. Cut butter into this mixture until crumbly (size of peas). Sprinkle the crumbly mixture over apples and bake for 35 to 40 minutes. Serve warm with vanilla ice cream.

Catherine Fong
Webb

LEMON ANGEL

SERVES: 8

Juice of 6 to 7 lemons
1 tablespoon gelatin
3 lemon rinds, grated
6 eggs, separated

1 heaping cup sugar
1 large angel food cake
Whipped cream

Heat juice until just hot. Dissolve gelatin in juice and cool. Beat juice mixture, rind, yolks and ½ cup sugar. In separate bowl, beat egg whites. Gradually add remaining sugar. Fold the two mixtures together in a large bowl. Break cake into small pieces. Fold cake into lemon mixture. Pour into 3 quart glass bowl. Refrigerate. Garnish with whipped cream, strawberries, and mint leaves.

Emily Cooper
Clarksdale

HOLIDAY DIVINITY

3 cups sugar
¾ cup white corn syrup
¾ cup water
1 teaspoon salt

2 egg whites
1 3-ounce package red or
   green gelatin
1 cup chopped pecans

Combine first four ingredients in heavy saucepan. Cook, on medium heat, to 252° on candy thermometer, stirring only until sugar is dissolved and mixture comes to a boil. Remove from heat. While above is cooking beat 2 egg whites to soft peaks. Gradually add gelatin, and continue beating. Slowly drip hot mixture into egg whites, beating at medium speed until it loses its gloss. Fold in pecans Drop by teaspoon on greased sheet or marble. Do not make if rainy. My mother always made this for my children at Christmas.

Eileen Massie Casburn
Sumner

BUTTERMILK PRALINES

YIELD: 40 TO 48

2 cups sugar
1 teaspoon soda
1 cup buttermilk

¾ cup butter or margarine
1 teaspoon vanilla
2 cups pecans

Combine all ingredients, except vanilla and pecans, in buttered large glass mixing bowl. Cover with plastic wrap (make a small hole in the plastic). Microwave on medium high for 15 minutes. Stir and continue cooking on medium high for 13 to 15 minutes or until a soft ball forms in cold water. Add vanilla and beat until mixture forms soft peaks. Stir in pecans. Pour spoonfuls on wax paper to cool.

Susan Connell
Clarksdale

CATHY'S FAMOUS CHRISTMAS FUDGE

I have been cooking this fudge for family and friends at Christmas since I was 12 years old. It always turns out great.

YIELD: 60

5 cups sugar
1 (12 ounce) can evaporated milk
1 (12 ounce) package semi-sweet chocolate morsels

¼ cup margarine
1 (7 ounce) jar marshmallow creme
1 cup chopped pecans

In a five quart heavy sauce pot, combine sugar and evaporated milk. Bring to a boil, reduce heat slightly and stirring constantly, boil 7 minutes. Remove from burner and stir in other ingredients. Pour into buttered 3 quart glass dish. When cool, cut into small squares. It's very rich and can be frozen.

Cathy Middleton
Clarksdale

SARA JANE'S TOFFEE

2 cups sugar
1 cup water
3 sticks butter - not
margarine

4½ cups finely chopped nuts
(pecans)
12 chocolate candy bars

Combine first three ingredients and bring to a boil until it reaches 280° on candy thermometer. Add 1½ cups nuts - continue cooking, stirring constantly until thermometer reaches 310°. Pour onto 2 greased cookie sheets quickly spreading 6 chocolate bars and then 1½ cups nuts over top side. Flip over and repeat using the other 6 chocolate bars and nuts.

Patsy Maclin
Clarksdale

HOT HERSHEY SANDWICH

This was the result of receiving a box of Hershey Bars and an electric sandwich grill one Christmas years ago. I wanted to use both gifts at the same time—voilà—the hot Hershey Sandwich! I have discovered that this is a favorite after school snack for French children.

YIELD: 1   OVEN: 400°

Butter two slices of bread on the outside. Place one Hershey Chocolate Bar in between. Place in electric sandwich grill for about 5 minutes. When the butter melts into the chocolate, the result is a delicious hot chocolate sandwich which will give you enough energy to see you through the day.

Mary Jo McIntosh
Clarksdale

MARY ANN CANDY

The lemon flavoring is the secret of this candy. We always make it at Christmas when all the children are home.

3 cups granulated sugar
1½ cups rich cream
½ teaspoon lemon flavoring

1½ ounces bitter chocolate, melted

Cook sugar and cream to a soft ball stage. Remove from stove. Over top put ½ teaspoon lemon flavoring. Do not stir. When almost cold, beat until it loses its gloss and becomes thick. Be sure to have several beaters, and do not use a mixer. Put in buttered 8 x 8 inch pan. When completely cool, spread over this the melted chocolate as thin as possible. When it hardens, cut into small squares.

Family Secret: Do not cook unless sunny!

Eileen M. Casburn
Sumner

PEANUT BUTTER BALLS

YIELD: 200

1 pound butter (or margarine)
3 pounds confectioner's sugar

2 pounds peanut butter
3 large packages semi-sweet chocolate chips
⅛ pound paraffin

Melt butter. Mix with sugar and peanut butter. Roll into small balls. Refrigerate 2 hours or more. Melt chocolate chips and paraffin. Dip the chilled balls into chocolate and place on waxed paper to set. (This is a great recipe for the Christmas holidays. Will keep for 6 weeks in refrigerator.)

Wanda Whaley
Clarksdale

VARIATION:
2 cups non-fat dry milk solids
1 cup wheat germ

1 cup peanut butter
1 cup corn syrup
½ cup margarine, melted

Mix all ingredients and proceed as indicated above.

Emily Cooper
Clarksdale

PECAN OR PEANUT BRITTLE

1 cup sugar
¾ cup white corn syrup
½ cup water
1 cup raw nuts (pecans or
  peanuts) (if using pecans
  chop coarsely or break
  them up)

1 teaspoon baking soda
1 teaspoon vanilla
1 teaspoon margarine

Mix sugar, water, and white corn syrup in a two quart heavy saucepan. Cook with candy thermometer to hard crack stage (takes about 10 minutes). Stir often. When sugar mixture reaches hard crack, (have all other ingredients measured out, in small pieces of aluminum foil), add raw nuts stirring constantly until sugar and nut mixture is a golden color. Quickly add soda, margarine, and vanilla (mixture will foam). Pour quickly onto buttered aluminum foil, and let cool, then break apart. Does not work well on a rainy day. Store in air-tight container.

Roselyn Dulaney
Clarksdale

THREE FRUIT SHERBET

SERVES: 12 TO 15

Juice of 3 oranges and 3
  lemons
3 bananas (mashed in
  blender or food processor)
1½ to 2 cups sugar
  (depending on tartness of
  fruit)

1 large instant vanilla
  pudding (6 ounces)
1 can sweetened condensed
  milk
Whole milk (enough to fill
  ice cream freezer can two-
  thirds full)

Mix juices and mashed bananas. Add sugar and set aside to let sugar dissolve. Mix dry pudding mix with sweetened condensed milk, then add to fruit mixture. Pour into one gallon freezer can and fill remainder of can with whole milk until two-thirds full. Freeze as usual.

Mrs. Hartley Kittle (Lynn)
Clarksdale

PEACH ICE CREAM

SERVES: 20 TO 25

⅓ cup flour
⅛ teaspoon salt
1½ cups sugar
10 eggs
1 quart milk, scalded
1 tablespoon vanilla
½ teaspoon dry ascorbic acid
   crystals
1 quart crushed peaches

1½ cups sugar
1 cup sour cream
2 teaspoons almond extract
1 pint whipping cream
1 (12 ounce) can evaporated
   milk
1 cup toasted finely chopped
   almonds (optional)

Make custard with first six ingredients; mix flour, sugar, and salt; beat in eggs, one or two at a time, and beat with wire whisk after each addition. Gradually add hot milk, beating while adding. Put mixture into double boiler and cook till mixture coats spoon. Cool, then add vanilla. Next, sprinkle ascorbic acid crystals over peaches. Add 1½ cups sugar, sour cream, and almond extract. Mix together. Pour custard into 1½ gallon freezer. Add peach mixture then add whipping cream and evaporated milk and almonds if you want them. Freeze, then pack. The custard and peaches can be prepared the day before.

Family Secret: This was the prize winning ice cream recipe at the Delta Jubilee in 1988. Use very ripe peaches if possible.

Harvey Fiser
Clarksdale

APRICOT ICE

SERVES: 8 TO 10

2½ cups orange juice,
   fresh or frozen
1½ cups sugar
1 cup water

¼ cup fresh lemon juice
Grated rind of 2 oranges
1 (21 ounce) can apricots,
   puréed

Make syrup of sugar and water. Add other ingredients. Mix well and freeze. Top with whipped cream and a maraschino cherry.

Baby Doll Peacock Waller (Mrs. Ben, Jr.)
Tribbett

ICE CREAM DESSERT

SERVES: 12

½ gallon vanilla ice cream, softened
3 tablespoons instant coffee
3 tablespoons hot water
6 chocolate covered toffee bars, frozen in wrappers

1 dozen lady fingers
1 pint whipping cream
3 tablespoons powdered sugar
3 tablespoons clear Crème de Cacao

Dissolve instant coffee in water. Mix with ice cream. With a hammer break candy in small pieces while still in wrapper. Add to ice cream mixture. Line springform pan with lady fingers. Fill with ice cream and freeze. Whip cream, adding sugar and Crème de Cacao. To serve: Remove from freezer several minutes before serving. Remove sides of pan. Slice dessert and top each serving with whipped cream.

Eva Connell
Clarksdale

STRAWBERRY ICE CREAM
(OR PEACH OR FRESH FIG)

SERVES: 12 TO 15

1½ cups of sugar
⅔ cup water
2 egg whites
1 quart sweetened mashed strawberries, peaches or figs

Few drops food coloring
Cream and milk, as desired

Beat egg whites until stiff. Cook sugar and water until it spins a thread. Pour cooked sugar water mixture over egg whites in small bowl of electric mixer. Beat at high speed until it reaches consistency of cake icing. Add this to the mashed, sweetened fruit. A couple of drops of red food coloring will pink the peaches or strawberries. Add enough heavy cream and milk to fill a gallon ice cream freezer two-thirds full. Freeze.

Matsy Shea
Dumas, Arkansas

CHOCOLATE GRAVY

3 cups boiling water
1 heaping tablespoon cocoa
2 heaping tablespoons flour
1 dash salt

½ to ¾ cup of sugar
(according to how sweet
you like it)

Bring water to a boil and keep it boiling. Mix all dry ingredients: Make sure no lumps. Place in saucepan on high heat. Pour in 1 cup boiling water, stir, stir. Then add the 2nd cup of boiling water. If it is too thick add ¼ cup more water. Let boil for 3 minutes. Stir all the time. This is very smooth chocolate sauce.

BISCUIT RECIPE FOR CHOCOLATE GRAVY:

2 cups flour
4 teaspoons baking powder
½ teaspoon salt

½ cup shortening
1 egg
⅔ cup milk

Mix dry ingredients, cut in shortening; stir in eggs and milk. Place on floured board. Knead 10 times. Roll and cut with 2½ inch cutter. Bake at 450° for 10 minutes.

Family Secret: Try this over hot biscuits for breakfast for an unusual treat!

Joan Ray
Tutwiler

JANE'S HOT FUDGE SAUCE

YIELD: 1½ TO 2 CUPS

2 cups sugar
1 (13 ounce) can evaporated
   milk
4 squares unsweetened
   chocolate

¼ cup butter
1 teaspoon vanilla

Put sugar and milk in 2 quart saucepan. Put on medium heat, bring to boil, stirring constantly. Let boil one minute. Add four squares chocolate, stirring until completely dissolved. Add butter and mix well. Let cool, then add vanilla. Store in refrigerator. When ready to use remove portion desired, warm in double boiler. Never boil it.

Mrs. Harris Barnes, Jr.
Clarksdale

LEMON SAUCE

YIELD: 1½ TO 2 CUPS

3 egg yolks	¾ cup sugar
Juice of 3 lemons	⅛ pound butter

Beat all ingredients together thoroughly and cook in double boiler until THICK! You may double amount.

Family Secret: This sauce is super over any plain white cake, pound cake, angel food, or cup cakes. Will keep in refrigerator. Also a good cake filling.

Gay Flowers
Dublin

PRALINE SAUCE

1½ cups light brown sugar	1 teaspoon vanilla
⅔ cup white corn syrup	1 cup chopped nuts
¼ cup or ½ stick butter	
1 (5¾ ounce) can evaporated milk	

Bring first three ingredients to a boil and let boil only about ½ minute. Let cool and add milk and vanilla. Whisk until smooth. Add nuts.

Family Secret: Delicious on ice cream.

Mrs. Ben Walker, Jr.
Tribbett

INDEX

INDEX

INDEX

COOKBOOK ORDER FORM

Family Secrets
Lee Academy
415 Lee Drive
Clarksdale, Mississippi 38614

Please send me _____ copies at $14.95 per copy plus $2.50 per copy for postage and handling. Enclosed is my check or money order for _____

_____
Name

_____
Address

_____
City and State   Zip Code

Mississippi residents add $1.05 per book for state sales tax.
Make checks payable to: Lee Academy.

- -

COOKBOOK ORDER FORM

Family Secrets
Lee Academy
415 Lee Drive
Clarksdale, Mississippi 38614

Please send me _____ copies at $14.95 per copy plus $2.50 per copy for postage and handling. Enclosed is my check or money order for _____

_____
Name

_____
Address

_____
City and State   Zip Code

Mississippi residents add $1.05 per book for state sales tax.
Make checks payable to: Lee Academy.

- -

COOKBOOK ORDER FORM

Family Secrets
Lee Academy
415 Lee Drive
Clarksdale, Mississippi 38614

Please send me _____ copies at $14.95 per copy plus $2.50 per copy for postage and handling. Enclosed is my check or money order for _____

_____
Name

_____
Address

_____
City and State   Zip Code

Mississippi residents add $1.05 per book for state sales tax.
Make checks payable to: Lee Academy.

Reorder Additional Copies

I would like to see **FAMILY SECRETS** in the following store in my area.

Store Name _____

Address _____

City _____ State _____ Zip _____

Store Name _____

Address _____

City _____ State _____ Zip _____

- -

I would like to see **FAMILY SECRETS** in the following store in my area.

Store Name _____

Address _____

City _____ State _____ Zip _____

Store Name _____

Address _____

City _____ State _____ Zip _____

- -

I would like to see **FAMILY SECRETS** in the following store in my area.

Store Name _____

Address _____

City _____ State _____ Zip _____

Store Name _____

Address _____

City _____ State _____ Zip _____